101 Thing
with Spare Moments
on the Ward

To Tina and Tony Evans, who have been both blessed and cursed by never having had a bored moment with nothing to do. Without them, this book would never have been written.

Dason Evans

To my wife, sister and parents for their everlasting love and support.

Nakul Gamanlal Patel

101 Things to Do with Spare Moments on the Ward

DASON E EVANS
MBBS(Lond), MHPE(Maastricht), fHEA
Honorary Senior Lecturer in Medical Education,
Barts and the London School of Medicine and Dentistry,
Queen Mary, University of London
Speciality Doctor in Sexual Health, St George's NHS Trust

NAKUL GAMANLAL PATEL
BSc(Hons), MBBS(Lond), MRCS(Eng)
Plastic Surgery Specialty Registrar East of England Deanery
Norfolk and Norwich University Hospitals NHS Foundation Trust
Addenbrooke's Hospital, Cambridge University Hospitals
NHS Foundation Trust
St Andrew's Centre for Plastic Surgery and Burns,
Broomfield Hospital, Mid Essex Hospital Services NHS Trust
Lister Hospital, East and North Hertfordshire NHS Trust

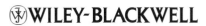

WILEY-BLACKWELL

A John Wiley & Sons, Ltd., Publication

Blackwell Publishing was acquired by John Wiley & Sons in February 2007. Blackwell's publishing program has been merged with Wiley's global Scientific, Technical and Medical business to form Wiley-Blackwell.

Registered office: John Wiley & Sons, Ltd, The Atrium, Southern Gate, Chichester, West Sussex, PO19 8SQ, UK

Editorial offices: 9600 Garsington Road, Oxford, OX4 2DQ, UK
The Atrium, Southern Gate, Chichester, West Sussex, PO19 8SQ, UK
111 River Street, Hoboken, NJ 07030-5774, USA

For details of our global editorial offices, for customer services and for information about how to apply for permission to reuse the copyright material in this book please see our website at www.wiley.com/wiley-blackwell.

Library of Congress Cataloging-in-Publication Data
Evans, Dason.
  101 things to do with spare moments on the ward / Dason E. Evans, Nakul Gamanlal Patel.
     p. ; cm.
  One hundred one things to do with spare moments on the ward
  One hundred and one things to do with spare moments on the ward
  Includes bibliographical references and index.
  ISBN-13: 978-1-4051-5985-2 (pbk. : alk. paper)
  ISBN-10: 1-4051-5985-5 (pbk. : alk. paper)
  I. Patel, Nakul Gamanlal.   II. Title.   III. Title: One hundred one things to do with spare moments on the ward.   IV. Title: One hundred and one things to do with spare moments on the ward.
  [DNLM: 1. Education, Medical.   2. Clinical Competence.   3. Learning.   W 18]
  LC-classification not assigned
  610.72'4–dc23

                              2011024776

A catalogue record for this book is available from the British Library.

Set in 8 on 10 pt Humanist Light by Toppan Best-set Premedia Limited
Printed and bound in Malaysia by Vivar Printing Sdn Bhd

1   2012

Contents

Foreword

This is an extraordinary book built around quotations from medical students and turned into a beautifully woven catalogue of learning opportunities around the ward. Walking to the wards to teach medical students, I often ask 'what did you learn yesterday?' The answer is often 'I went home as the teaching was cancelled and there was nothing to do'. A source of great sadness to me and, dare I say it, almost equivalent to a child saying 'I am bored' with the hidden implication of '. . . entertain me'. There is just so much going on in both the hospital and primary care settings that I am often left speechless. But, was I too harsh in my judgement? If students did not know what the learning opportunities were, or indeed, how to find them, then their reply to me was hardly surprising.

This book aims to redress this gap and made me realise that my irritation was, indeed, harsh. It carefully points out the opportunities available but often so invisible to a young student's inexperienced eye. Quietly surveying the hive of activity from the end of a ward makes it easier to spot points of interest, almost like a game – the nurses giving out medications, pharmacists doing chart rounds, doctors doing ward rounds, the social worker enquiring about the domestic situations of patients about to be discharged, the ECG technician or junior doctor doing an ECG, the F1 doctor looking at an X-ray, and above all, patients lying in bed dying for someone to chat to them about their condition or just about anything! All useful opportunities that cannot be learned from textbooks, but which could make the learning easier with practical examples from real life.

What I liked most about this book is that the suggestions for these learning opportunities came mostly from medical students themselves. They had discovered them on their own and were passing them onto other student colleagues as suggestions for that spare moment that should not be wasted! The chapters address communication, examination and procedures to prescribing, data interpretation and how to motivate people to actually teach you. A host of useful hints and suggestions set out in a most readable way and suggested by student peers. Suggestions that you could follow up alone, or indeed learn in a two-way conversation with a friend.

I think this book will certainly have a niche in the texts available for students to buy. It is well set out, eminently readable and, fun! There is so much to learn and so little time to do so, so why not spend it on the wards and learn from clinical practise? The authors of this book tell you how!

Parveen J Kumar CBE, MD, FRCP, FRCPE, FRCPath
Professor of Medicine and Education
Barts and the London School of Medicine and Dentistry
Queen Mary, University of London
London

Abbreviations and Medical hierarchy

Abbreviations

A&E	– Accident and Emergency
ABG	– Arterial Blood Gas
ABPI	– Ankle–Brachial Pressure Index
Abx	– Antibiotic
ADL	– Activities of Daily Living
AFP	– α-Fetoprotein
AIDS	– Acquired Immune Deficiency Syndrome
BBB	– Bundle Branch Block
BMA	– British Medical Association
BMJ	– British Medical Journal
BNF	– British National Formulary
BP	– Blood Pressure
BPM	– Beats Per Minute
COPD	– Chronic Obstructive Pulmonary Disease
CT	– Computerised Tomography
CTPA	– Computerised Tomography Pulmonary Angiogram
ECG	– Electrocardiogram
ERCP	– Endoscopic Retrograde Cholangiopancreatography
EWTD	– European Working Time Directive
FBC	– Full Blood Count
U&Es	– Urea and Electrolytes
GALS	– Gait, Arms, Legs, Spine examination
GI	– Gastrointestinal
GP	– General Practitioner
HAI	– Hospital-Acquired Infection
HR	– Heart Rate
IM	– Intramuscular
INR	– International Normalised Ratio
ITU	– Intensive Therapy Unit
IV	– Intravenous
IVP	– Intravenous Pyelogram
JVP	– Jugular Venous Pressure
MAU	– Medical Assessment Unit
MDT	– Multidisciplinary Team

MI   – Myocardial Infarction
MRI   – Magnetic Resonance Imaging
MRSA   – Methicillin-Resistant Staphylococcus Aureus
NG   – Nasogastric
NHS   – National Health Service
NPSA   – National Patient Safety Association
NSAID   – Non-Steroidal Anti-Inflammatory Drug
OGD   – Oesophago-Gastro-Duodenoscopy
OSCE   – Objective Structured Clinical Exam
PACS   – Picture Archive and Communication System
PALS   – Patient Liaison Service
PE   – Pulmonary Embolus
PMH   – Past Medical History
PPE   – Peer Physical Examination
RPM   – Rate Per Minute
RR   – Respiratory Rate
SALT   – Speech And Language Therapy
SSC   – Student-Selected Component
STEMI   – ST-Elevation Myocardial Infarction
STI   – Sexually Transmitted Infection
TEDS   – Thromboembolic Deterrent Stockings
WHO   – World Health Organisation

Medical hierarchy

Pre MMC Training System	Post MMC Training System	Outside Commonwealth
PRHO	F1 or FY1	Intern or First-Year Resident
SHO	F2 or FY2	Resident up to Chief Resident
SHO	ST1	
SHO	ST2	
REG/SPR/STR	ST3 up to ST9	
CON	CON	Attending

CON   – Consultant
F1 or FY1 – Foundation Year 1
MMC   – Modernising Medical Careers
PRHO   – Preregistration House Officer
REG   – Registrar
SHO   – Senior House Officer
ST3   – Specialist Training Year 3
STR   – Specialty Registrar
SPR   – Specialist Registrar

Introduction

The idea behind this book was born some years ago, when one of the authors was talking to a tutee. When asked about what he had done the day before he said:

I went home early, as teaching was cancelled, nothing was happening and I was bored.

On talking to other students and, indeed, from our own recollection of medical school, this was clearly a common phenomenon. This student was surrounded by possibilities for learning, but didn't see any of them; nothing was happening. This anecdote is not, in any way, meant as a criticism of this student, or even students in general; it is just the way that things are. It was thanks to this student that the idea of this book was formed.

In this book, students, medical school staff, hospital staff and a wide range of other people from around the world have submitted ideas for 'things to do' when students might find themselves 'bored' or 'with spare moments' in the clinical environment. We took hundreds of suggestions, tried to cluster them into themes, and clustered the themes into sections including teaching, testing and learning, clinical communication, physical examination, practical procedures and a host of other topics.

This book has two aims. First, it gives a list of possibilities for 'things to do' when nothing seems to be happening. These possibilities were submitted by students and staff who have been in exactly this situation, so these ideas represent tried and tested opportunities for learning. We have tried to make the book small enough to fit in a pocket, and have given various different ways of accessing the task (see below in 'How to use this book'), to make it as easy as possible to find an inspiring idea of something to do that fits with your mood of the moment.

The second aim is a little more subtle: we hope that this book not only gives you a list of things to do, but will also help you spot other opportunities around you, will help you to try out these opportunities and will encourage you to share these with others. To this aim we have included lots of suggestions for 'taking things further' and have tried to select suggestions and a commentary that highlight some of the skills that will make your life easier – giving it a go, dealing with rejection, utilising 'cheek and charm'.

How to use this book

We would recommend that you read this introduction before starting, particularly this section, and the section on 'What you will need' and 'A word on professionalism' – these apply to the whole book. After that, it's really up to you. We have written the book in such a way that you can start at the front and work your way through, or you can dip in and out to sections that seem relevant to you *today*. We imagine that, if dipping in, you will find the table of contents (which lists all the themes in each section), and also the table of tasks useful (page xix). The latter contains icons that allow the student to quickly spot possible tasks that will fit with their mood, availability of people and time.

This is not, of course, a book for the bookshelf. Flick through it in spare moments, highlight ideas that you want to try, keep it handy on the wards, on the bus, add your own ideas – just not in the library copy!

For students

This is not the kind of book that you will have seen before. There are plenty of textbooks for medicine, loads of exam guides and cramming books; one or two books on how to study at medical school, but nothing quite like this.

Professor Geoff Norman is a well-known Canadian medical educationalist; he specialises in the topic of the development of medical expertise (he is an expert in expertise, if you will, which has to be a niche market!) and in a keynote lecture at a large medical education conference a few years ago he reviewed the literature on the development of expertise. It takes 10 years, roughly 10 000 hours of deliberate, reflective practice to become an expert. He asked the audience what the expert gets from these 10 years of experience, and answered '10 years worth of experienc**es**'. This book aims to help you fill spare moments with experiences that will help you become a better doctor, and also help you enjoy your studies. All those spare 10 minutes, half-hours and half-days add up.

What you will need
We suggest that you need a couple of simple things in addition to this book to get the most out of it. You probably have them already.

A **diary** is a must for a clinical medical student, or at the least a timetable with the next month ahead planned out. Imagine that you pop down to the ECG department (Task 43) when teaching has been cancelled, but they can't take you then. They are impressed at how keen you are and ask if you can make it in 2 weeks' time – you need to quickly know when you might be free. Similarly you might put in your diary to look up a patient's results or find out how they did in theatre, or even read about the anatomy of the thyroid the night before theatre next week (Tasks 7 and 88). A diary puts you in control. If you don't have one, now is the time to buy one!

You will also need a **notebook**. Many of the suggestions require a little bit of follow-up, or maybe some ongoing discussion with your colleagues; you will need a notebook that is small enough to fit in your pocket and large enough to have a separate page or two for each task. If you like stationery as much as us, then spend some time finding something that you like – perhaps with different colour sections. Start one section, perhaps right in the centre of the book, to write down your own ideas for things that students could do in their spare moments. Try them out, share them with others and even consider submitting them at **www.101things.org**.

We suggest that you keep some kind of **Portfolio** to keep track of your learning. If you school does not give you one, or if you do not find their's useful, why not create your own?

A word on ethics and professionalism

It is necessary to highlight that these submissions were written with some fundamental premises in mind, and these are so fundamental that they are often not mentioned explicitly:

- **Informed consent is mandatory**. Your role in the clinical environment is to learn, and patients must know this so that they can freely decide whether or not to give the gift of their consent. The good news is that most patients are more than happy to help students learn. Your medical school will have formal teaching and expectations around consent, and it is also covered in books such as *How to Succeed at Medical School* (Evans and Brown, 2009 pp. 47–8) and the BMA's *Medical Ethics* today (English et al. 2004).

- **You should be competent enough** at whatever you practise. Some of the suggestions, e.g. practising phlebotomy, require a degree of competency to practise with patients or peers even when supervised. Clearly you should do these tasks only if you are competent enough. Some tasks in the book will be suitable for first year medical students, others will not.

- You should ensure that you have **adequate supervision** for whatever tasks you are practising. If looking through the equipment cupboard to see what you do and don't recognise (Task 36) this might be as simple as just asking the nurses if that's OK, but if rewriting a medication chart (Task 53) for the first time then you want to make pretty sure that someone will supervise and check your work thoroughly.

- **Knowing when to stop** can sometimes not be as simple as it might sound. The patient might say 'Don't worry, have [yet] another go at taking blood', but if you suspect that you are beginning to abuse their generosity, you probably are.

- **Knowing when not to start** can also be tricky for the enthusiastic student. Be aware of the climate. If the nurses are fuming after a heated exchange with one of the doctors or matron or an angry relative, now might not be the best time to ask them to show you how to set up an intravenous line, but, if you know them well enough, it might be a good time to offer to go and take patients' observations for them.

For staff

The clinical learning environment is changing; patients are spending less time in hospital, and tend to be more ill while they are there. Changes resulting from the

European Working Time Directorate (EWTD) have resulted in a degradation of the traditional firm structure, prohibiting some of the educational relationships between students and juniors on the firms that used to be common (Spencer 2003; Nikendei et al. 2006). In addition, there has been a shift in clinical medicine toward more explicit accountability, job planning and formal outcome measures, which has affected the delicate balance of service, teaching and research (the 'three-legged stool' after Weisbord 1985).

In reaction to these challenges to clinical learning, some authors have called for students to spend less time on the wards, and more time in simulation, learning from manikins, computers and role-play. In this book we offer an alternative solution. We believe passionately that medicine is learnt with and from patients, and we have seen clearly that some students thrive in the clinical learning environment, seeking out varied learning opportunities that will help them develop into skilled and experienced junior doctors. This book aims to take the best tips from those students and staff, and share them with others, encouraging all students to make the very best use of those opportunities around them.

Staff, whether clinicians who teach or medical school staff, may find this text useful, both for giving students ideas on how to fill spare moments productively, and also for helping students to learn to spot those opportunities themselves. If you are the consultant or trainee with responsibility for students on attachment, why not start a book or folder of opportunities available while on attachment with your team, and encourage the students to take responsibility for adding new opportunities to the book as they arise and useful notes for the next set of students coming ('Fridays are a bad day for the ECG department, try to go down on any day other than a Friday!').

If you find some suggestions missing from this book, then please highlight these to your students, and even consider making a submission to **www.101things.org**.

References

English V, Sommerville A, British Medical Association (2004). *Medical Ethics Today: The BMA's handbook of ethics and law*. London: BMJ Books.

Evans D, Brown J (2009). *How to Succeed at Medical School: An essential guide to learning*. Oxford: Wiley-Blackwell.

Nikendei C, Kraus B, Schrauth M, Weyrich P, Zipfel S, Junger J (2006). An innovative model for final-year students' skills training course in internal medicine: 'essentials from admission to discharge'. *Med Teach* **28**:648–51.

Spencer J (2003). Learning and teaching in the clinical environment. *BMJ* **326**:591–4.

Weisbord MR (1985). Overall diagnosis: building a profile [1]. A diagnostic profile [2]. In: *Organizational Diagnosis: A workbook of theory and practice. Health Care Management Review 1, 2*. Addison-Wesley Publishing Co.

Acknowledgements

This book is unusual, perhaps unique, within medical education in its approach. The contents of the book are written by people just like you, students and staff who know that, at times, you can have bored or quiet moments when you are in the clinical environment. As authors we have clustered these submissions, selected the ones that seemed most useful, most interesting or at times even most amusing, and joined them together with some commentary. For this book, therefore, the largest acknowledgement must go to these people who submitted ideas for the book – the wealth of ideas and information that are collected between these covers is thanks to their enthusiasm, innovation and willingness to share.

We have listed all the contributors below, and also in the text when we quote them directly. It should be noted that sometimes many contributors suggested the same or a very similar idea. In these cases we have chosen one that seemed to be the most representative. In these cases we have not directly acknowledged the others who have suggested similar ideas, because this would have taken a lot of space and been rather dull to read. In listing the contributors below, we thank and acknowledge them for all of their submissions, whether they have been directly quoted or not.

Of course there are some people who we would like to particularly thank for their input into this book. Abigail Cole, a medical student at St George's, University of London had a large input into writing the first section, and we thank her for her speed, efficiency and for the fantastic section. Catherine Joekes, lecturer in clinical communication at St George's, University of London, was kind enough to read and critique earlier drafts of the section on clinical communication and give incredibly useful feedback, for which we are very grateful. Ammy Lam, Principal Pharmacist at Barts and the London NHS Trust, gave invaluable advice and insight for the section on prescribing including an innovative way to learn about medication errors. Barts and the London NHS Trust have also given their formal permission to use their medication cards for our examples, allowing us to make these examples as real as possible. Andrew Webb, Senior Lecturer/Honorary Consultant in Clinical Pharmacology at Kings College London and Clinical Pharmacology at St Thomas' Hospital, London gave us permission to use his innovative way to thing about medicines – 'Use your BRAINS before you AIMS'.

As this book represented such an innovative approach to publishing for medical education we have to thank Wiley-Blackwell for their support, particularly Martin Sugden, our commissioning editor, whose passion, enthusiasm and vision seemed to know no bounds. Elizabeth Johnston and Laura Murphy have looked after us during the long and complex process of working out the right way to present this book. This was a new process for all of us and, although we have tested their patience to the limit, their constructive advice and support have been invaluable.

Of course, the most useful feedback has come from a wide body of people, including some fantastic student reviewers for Wiley-Blackwell, and too many friends, colleagues and students to mention by name – we appreciate you all!

Below, we have listed the details that were right at the time that the contributors submitted their ideas, we realise that people have graduated, moved and may even have changed their names since then. As an aside, this book started as a project called '101 things to do on the wards when bored' and has subsequently been renamed. We mention this only because a significant number of the submissions, from both students and staff, mention being 'bored', and we would like to clarify that this is a reflection of the initial title of the project, rather than any reflection on the attitude of those who submitted the ideas.

List of contributors

May Abboudi, Medical Student, King's College London, UK

Ziena Abdullah, Medical Student, Barts and The Royal, London, UK

Ravi Agarwal, Medical Student, Barts and The Royal, London, UK

Ravi Agarwal, Medical Student, Barts and The Royal, London, UK

Kumar Ahuja, Medical Student, Barts and The Royal, London, UK

Ijeoma Akunna, Medical Student, King's College London, UK

Hussain Al-Hashimi, Medical Student, St George's Medical School, UK

Mosaab Aljalahma, Medical Student, University of Glasgow, Kuwait

Ali Al-Lami, Medical Student, Barts and The Royal, London, UK

Omayma Aly, Doctor, Cairo, Egypt

Linzi Arkus, Medical Student, St George's Medical School, UK

Donna Arya, Medical Student, Barts and The Royal, London, UK

Gaurav Asal, Medical Student, Barts and The Royal, London, UK

Rachelle Asciak, Medical Student, Mater Dei hospital, Malta

Anushka Aubeelack, Medical Student, Barts and The Royal, London, UK

Fenella Beynon, Medical Student, Imperial College London, UK

Savraj Bhangra, Medical Student, Barts and The Royal, London, UK

Asheesh Bharti, Medical Student, Barts and The London NHS Trust, UK

Ruth Bird, Medical Student, Barts and The Royal, London, UK

Sharon Bone, Medical Student, Barts and The Royal, London, UK

Alison Bradley, Medical Student, University of Dundee, UK

Daniel Braunold, Medical Student, Barts and The Royal, London, UK

Paul Cacciottolo, Medical Student, University of Malta Medical School, Malta

Junaid Campwala, Medical Student, Barts and The Royal, London, UK

Rebekah Carter, Staff Nurse, Broomfield Hospital, UK

Omar Chehab, Medical Student, Barts and The Royal London, UK

Shin Chia, Medical Student, Barts and The Royal, London, Malaysia

Emily Chung, Medical Student, Barts and The Royal, London, UK

Laura Cohen, Medical Student, St George's Medical School, UK

Catherine Connew, Staff Nurse, Broomfield Hospital, UK

Emma Court, Medical Student, Barts and The Royal, London, UK

Peter Cowell, Chaplain, Barts and The London NHS Trust, UK

Catherine Culley, Doctor, Brighton, UK

Karl Cutajar, Medical Student, Mater Dei hospital, Malta

Debi Dasgupta, Medical Student, Barts and The London NHS Trust, UK

Duncan Davidson, Medical Student, Columbia, USA

Almas Dawood, Medical Student, St George's Medical School, UK

Hareen De Silva, Medical Student, Barts and The Royal, London, UK

Katharine Elliott, Medical Student, University of Warwick, UK

Joanne Evans, Medical Student, Barts and The Royal, London, UK

Saleem Farooqui, Medical Student, St George's Medical School, UK

Asma Fazlanie, Medical Student, University of Sheffield, UK

Wee Fu Gan, Medical Student, Barts and The Royal, London, Malaysia

Laura Geddes, Medical Student, Barts and The Royal, London, UK

Rohit Ghurye, Medical Student, Brighton and Sussex Medical School, UK

Anna Green, Doctor, Royal Free Hospital, UK

Caris Grimes, Doctor, London, UK

Sameer Gujral, Clinical Teaching Fellow, Barts and The Royal, London, UK

Sophia Haywood, Work Experience Student, Norfolk & Norwich University Hospital, UK

Ruth Heseltine, Medical Student, Barts and The Royal, London, UK

Su Ping Hi, Medical Student, Edinburgh University, UK

Louise Holmqvist, Medical Student, Barts and The Royal, London, UK

Nazia Hossain, Medical Student, Barts and The Royal, London, UK

Sue Howarth, Medical Student, Barts and The Royal, London, UK

Sabih Momenhul Huq, Senior Lecturer, Barts and The London NHS Trust, UK

Anna Jenkins, Medical Student, St George's Medical School, UK

Amanda Jewison, Medical Student, Brighton and Sussex Medical School, UK

Sharavanan Jeyanathan, Medical Student, Barts and The Royal, London, UK

Daniel Jodocy, Medical Student, Medical University Innsbruck, Austria

Laura Kendal, Medical Student, King's College London, UK

San Khine, Medical Student, University of West Indies, Jamaica

Saw Sian Khoo, Doctor, Kuala Lumpur, Malaysia, Malaysia

Indrajith Kowarthanan, Medical Student, Barts and The Royal, London, UK

Ammy Lam, Senior Pharmacist, Barts and The London NHS Trust, UK

Germaine Leunissen, Doctor, Erasmus, NL

Sian Loae, Medical Student, Leicester University, UK

Wei Yang Low, Medical Student, Barts and The Royal, London, UK

Michael Magro, Medical Student, Barts and The Royal, London, UK

Viyaasan Mahalingasivam, Medical Student, Barts and The Royal, London, UK

Saima Mahmood, Doctor, St George's Medical School, UK

Angela McGilloway, Medical Student, Barts and The Royal, London, UK

Ronan McGinty, Doctor, Newcastle, UK

Martina Michels, Physiotherapist, SSMT Lugano, Switzerland

Fazia Mir, Doctor, Aga Khan University, Pakistan

Afrah Mohammed, Medical Student, Eastern Province Dammam, Saudi Arabia

Martin Mueller, Doctor, King's College London, UK

Lyndsey Muntane, Medical Student, Barts and The Royal, London, UK

Sameer Nakedar, Medical Student, Barts and The Royal, London, Zimbabwe

Ying Ci Ngg, Medical Student, Barts and The Royal, London, UK

Eimear O'Connor, Medical Student, University of Glasgow, UK

Amit Odelia, Medical Student, Barts and The Royal, London, UK

Nkem Okolo, Doctor, King's College Hospital, UK

Sarah Onida, Medical Student, King's College London, UK

Ravinder Pabla, Doctor, Broomfield Hospital, UK

Gaman Patel, Businessman, Leicester, UK

Hinesh Patel, Medical Student, Keele Medical School, UK

Kayur Patel, Medical Student, Imperial College London, UK

Meera Patel, Dentist and Author, Leicester, UK

Sameer Patel, Medical Student, Brighton and Sussex Medical School, UK

Sangita Patel, Teacher, Leicester, UK

Sheetal Patel, Senior Economic Consultant, London, UK

Sabra Pechrak-Manesh, Medical Student, Barts and The Royal, London, UK

Andrew Pelham, Medical Student, Barts and The Royal, London, UK

Jennifer Pennekett, Medical Student, Barts and The Royal, London, UK

Sarah Perkin, Medical Student, St George's Medical School, UK

Natasa Perovic, Learning Technologist, Barts and The Royal, London, UK

Donna Pilkington, Medical Student, Manchester University, UK

Ivana Pogledic, Doctor, University of Zagreb, Croatia

Tim Powell, Medical Student, St George's Medical School, UK

Abigail Randall, Medical Student, Barts and The Royal, London, UK

David Randall, Medical Student, Barts and The Royal, London, UK

Devina Raval, Medical Student, Barts and The Royal, London, UK

Bhavin Rawal, Medical Student, Barts and The Royal, London, UK

Shmuel Reis, Head of Medical Education, Technion, Haifa, Israel

Ben Rhodes, Chaplain, Barts and The London NHS Trust, UK

Kathryn Rhodes, Medical Student, St George's Medical School, UK

Michael Richardson, Medical Student, Manchester University, UK

Anneka Rose, Medical Student, St George's Medical School, UK

Nabila Salahuddin, Medical Student, Barts and The Royal, London, UK

Charity Santeng, Medical Student, Barts and The Royal, London, UK

Maria See, Medical Student, Barts and The Royal, London, UK

Claire Seeley, Medical Student, Barts and The Royal, London, UK

Emma Short, Medical Student, Barts and The Royal, London, UK

Ashley Simpson, Medical Student, Barts and The Royal, London, UK

Klaudine Simpson, Senior Clinical Skills Tutor, Cambridge University, UK

Andrew Smith, Medical Student, Barts and The London NHS Trust, UK

Carmen Eynon Soto, Medical Student, Barts and The Royal, London, UK

Simon Stallworthy, Medical Student, Barts and The Royal, London, UK

Amit Sunder, Dentist, Birmingham, UK

Asil Tahir, Medical Student, Barts and The Royal, London, UK

Sabrina Talukdar, Medical Student, Cambridge University, UK

Daijun Tan, Medical Student, Barts and The Royal, London, UK

Devangi Thakkar, Medical Student, Barts and The Royal, London, UK

Nhan Vo Thanh, Doctor and Teacher, University of Medicine and Pharmacy, Vietnam

Christopher Thexton, Medical Student, University of Glasgow, UK

Elizabeth Tissingh, Doctor, Belford Hospital, UK

Rima Vaid, Medical Student, Barts and The Royal, London, UK

Jolien Van Den Houten, Occupational Therapist, Zuyd University, The Netherlands

Canh Van On, Medical Student, King's College London, UK

Nupur Verma, Medical Student, Miami, USA

Thorrmela Vijayaseelan, Medical Student, St George's Medical School, UK

Umar Wali, Medical Student, St George's Medical School, UK

Andy Wearn, Clinical Senior Lecturer, Auckland, New Zealand

Andrew Webb, Senior Lecturer/ Honorary Consultant in Cardiovascular Clinical Pharmacology, Kings College London/ Guy's and St Thomas' NHS Trust UK

Mei Teng Wong, Medical Student, Barts and The Royal, London, UK

In appreciation of those making submissions, we held a prize draw, and Professor Parveen Kumar has selected the four winners though random allocation, who will each receive a free copy of this book. The winner's names are:

| Winner 1 | Mosaab Aljalahma | Winner 2 | Emma Court |
| Winner 3 | Rebekah Carter | Winner 4 | Viyaasan Mahalingasivam |

Table of tasks

Key to icons

Person

Patient

Professional (e.g. doctor, nurse)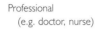

Peer

Combination

None

You

Time

Moments

Minutes

Hours

Ongoing

Variable

Task no.	Page number	Idea	Person	Time
Section 1 Teaching, Testing and Learning				
1	Page 3	Creating memory aids – mnemonics, diagrams and poems		
2	Page 4	Look into the origin of medical terms and diseases		
3	Page 5	Create a crossword		
4	Page 5	Radiological quiz		
5	Page 6	Study using flash cards		

Section 1
TEACHING, TESTING AND LEARNING

Co-Authored by Abigail Cole

You learn something every day if you pay attention.

Ray LeBlond

Introduction

The main purpose of being at medical school is to learn. This learning includes a huge amount of knowledge, a wide range of skills (including high-order thinking skills such as clinical reasoning) and the attitudes consistent with being a medical professional. This whole book is focused on learning in the clinical learning environment, of course, but the first section specifically clusters together some submissions, giving a range of different approaches to learning in your spare moments on the wards.

Most of the submissions in this section relate to learning knowledge. Clearly there is overlap with other sections, and we have cross-referenced to highlight this e.g. with the prescribing and data interpretation sections.

The themes within this section include reading around patients whom you see, suggestions involving mnemonics and memory aids, a wide variety of different approaches to quizzes and testing yourself and others, and some suggestions for e-learning/useful websites. These suggestions are not exhaustive. We hope that they will be useful and, indeed, that they may act as a trigger for you to find even more approaches. We have to note that, although the references were correct at the time of going to press, by the time you read this some of the web addresses may be out of date; if so, we have no doubt that you will be able to find and evaluate similar sources.

As people interested in education of medical students, we would like to reflect on some themes that run through these submissions, and some that are less evident. One of the most important concepts that comes through these submissions loud and clear is that of 'active learning', which is a widely used term with various definitions. At its most basic level it involves the student actively engaging with the learning material. This engagement usually, but not always, involves a peer and includes debating, teaching, testing, reorganising information, linking it with other learnt information, and manipulating it and applying it to new contexts. As a concept it contrasts nicely with more 'passive' approaches, such as trying to soak up information by sitting in a lecture and reading the words of a book without actually digesting the contents or the meaning. If you would like to read more, the article by John Spencer (1999) under

101 Things to Do with Spare Moments on the Ward, First Edition. Dason E Evans, Nakul Gamanlal Patel.
© 2012 Dason E Evans and Nakul Gamanlal Patel. Published 2012 by Blackwell Publishing Ltd.

Further reading is a good start, and there are plenty of study skills books for higher education (a number of good ones by Stella Cottrell, Tony Buzan and one specifically for medical students by Dason Evans and Jo Brown are listed in Further reading).

There is a great deal of evidence that active learning results in deeper learning – which includes both a better understanding and also better recall of the information learnt. So it is worthwhile thinking about your education and ensuring that you have an active approach. Many of the submissions in this section use peers to ensure active learning (through quizzes, explaining, 'doing', presenting, etc.), and many of the approaches are innovative and fun. Some approaches will be useful on those days when you are feeling more solitary.

Summary

The vast amount of knowledge that you will need to learn as a medical student and a doctor can be daunting. This section provides practical suggestions from other students, graduates and teaching staff on how to learn effectively and efficiently, ensuring active learning and with attention to your own motivation and having fun.

Theme: memory aids and mnemonics

Background

A widely accepted theory, proposed in the 1950s by George A Millar, was that short-term memory can process only seven units of information at any one time. Memory aids work by grouping these units of information, and associating them with an easy to remember word or poem. Often these associations are aided through being humorous, exaggerated or absurd, or with a sexual connotation, because these concepts are easier to remember!

Practising the ability to recall information is obviously key to performing well in exams. However, even in a ward setting, being able to recall information, e.g. the causes of pancreatitis (I GET SMASHED – **I**diopathic, **G**allstones, **E**thanol, **T**rauma, **S**teroids, **M**umps, **A**utoimmune disease, **S**corpion stings, **H**ypercalcaemia/**h**yperlipidaemia, **E**RCP, **D**rugs) can help aid diagnosis and treatment of a patient, and is well worth getting to grips with early on in your career. Everyone learns information in different ways: although one person may prefer visual representations, another may associate medical terms with a poem; the wide variety of suggestions compiled in this section may be of use to you, but the list is not exhaustive. There are many websites out there where you can find the type of learner that you are, and they make suggestions for the best way in which you may study.

Requirements

Something that you wish to recall, and a piece of paper to write your mnemonics down.

1. Creating memory aids — mnemonics, diagrams and poems

Creating your own memory aids has benefits in both the creating process by which you have to revise your knowledge and being able to use them later on as a device to recall facts.

When revising for exams we try to make our own funny medical mnemonics and try to teach these to our friends. These can be along the same as those that are commonly used in medicine/surgery in different contexts. They can be used throughout medical education, e.g. in anatomy a mnemonic for the carpal bones that I was taught:

~ Some   ~ Scaphoid
~ Lovers   ~ Lunate
~ Try   ~ Triquetrum
~ Positions   ~ Pisiform
~ That   ~ Trapezium
~ They   ~ Trapezoid
~ Can't   ~ Capitate
~ Handle   ~ Hamate

Rohit Ghuyre, Medical Student, UK

Note

1. If you don't wish to create your own mnemonics, some medical mnemonic books are available.

There are some good mnemonic aids available that are light to carry and can be used for quick revision. Why not flip to the relevant chapter to the rotation you are on and test your colleagues out! This will widen your knowledge and rather than read it yourself puts you on the spot.

Laura Geddes, Medical Student, UK

You could make pictures/doodles that would help remind you of a particular pattern of clinical signs, e.g. a picture of a cat's face might serve as a memory aid to remember which signs to look for during the obstetric exam.

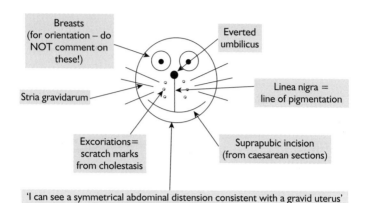

Breasts (for orientation – do NOT comment on these!)

Everted umbilicus

Stria gravidarum

Linea nigra = line of pigmentation

Excoriations= scratch marks from cholestasis

Suprapubic incision (from caesarean sections)

'I can see a symmetrical abdominal distension consistent with a gravid uterus'

Gaurav Semar, Medical Student, UK

Common diseases including their signs and symptoms and management are put in the form of poetry so that we can recall them quickly. We sit in a ring and write the signs and symptoms, investigations and treatment outlines. Then each one tries to put each item into a phrase and the other completes it ... then we take all our contributions and formulate them into one coherent poem which collates all about the disease.

Omayma Aly, Doctor, Egypt

2. Look into the origin of medical terms and diseases

By researching the origin of medical terms this may help relate the words with literal meanings. An example of this is 'diabetes' meaning 'a siphon'. Greek physician, Aretus the Cappadocian, named the condition 'diabetes' and explained that patients with it had polyuria and 'passed water like a siphon'. Knowing the etymology may help to recall this knowledge later on, when put on the spot and asked 'what is ... ?'.

Look up the etymology of medical terms — helps remember what they mean.

Duncan Davidson, Medical Student, Columbia

Taking it a step further

Look up the names of eponymous syndromes, i.e. who is Paget? How about Wilson of Wilson's disease? You will find some excellent books on medical eponyms in the library that make easier reading than the internet.

Theme: building quizzes

Background

Repetition is essential for the process of learning to take place. However, sometimes this process can feel tedious, and you may become demotivated, making it difficult to learn. Having more interesting ways to revise material can help improve your learning process. 'Quizzes' can come in all shapes and sizes, and vary from fun 'game' such as exercises, to more traditional question-and-answer-type structures. Quizzes focus on active learning, and require the learner to become engaged in thinking about the task. This may done as part of a group, or you may prefer to study alone; the tasks suggested in the section can be manipulated to suit the way in which you learn best.

Requirements

Material that you wish to revise.

3. Create a crossword

One can play a quiz concerning a crossword for medical terms and parts of human body in different languages.

Ivana Pogledic, Doctor, Croatia

Notes

1. Creating a crossword could be used to learn any material relevant to you.

2. If creating your own crossword is too time-consuming, there are lots of online resources for medical crosswords and other games. Try **www.doctorslounge.com** and search on their website for crosswords. For more e-learning suggestions see the theme 'e-learning resources' in this chapter.

3. For those more technologically minded, you will find plenty of software downloads and websites that will help you construct crosswords or word searches from lists of words.

4. Radiological quiz

Testing yourself and/or others on radiology is really easy with the availability of lots of different images in the hospital catalogues. Make sure that you look only at patients' pictures that are relevant to you or your colleague.

One can play a 5-minute quiz concerning MRI or CT images of different parts of human body.

Ivana Pogledic, Doctor, Croatia

Taking it a step further

1. As a group look at a radiograph and separately write down your observations and ultimately a diagnosis. Each discusses what he or she thought and why, and then confirms this with the radiographer's report. Make a note of anything that you didn't observe on the radiograph, to remember to look out for this next time.

2. Create a template of things that you will look at on a radiograph based on headings, i.e. time, date, rotation, penetration, airways, lung fields, etc. Use this as a checklist for you and colleagues to base your presentation. When quizzing each other on presenting the image, do you comment on all the areas of the template?

See also
Other suggestions around imaging, including Tasks 82 onwards.

5. Study using flash cards

Look up drug names and learn why they are used etc. If you make flashcards these can be carried in your pocket and turned over for the use/drug class and action from the name.

Ruth Bird, Medical Student, UK

Carry Gray's Anatomy flashcards around with you at all times. Use any 'empty' time to quiz your clinical partner on any aspect of anatomy. In 10 minutes you'll be surprised how much you can learn.

Laura Kendal, Medical Student, UK

Taking it a step further

1. Flash cards can be made to have any information on them that you want to learn. Why not create some for signs and symptoms of diseases.

Improve your knowledge of skin lesions — Carry flash cards or images on your phone of common skin lesions (benign and malignant). Most patients, particularly the elderly, will have at least one skin lesion. Try to identify the lesion by taking a quick history and examination. If you come across something you cannot classify this could lead to a further learning opportunity, through independent research. You may even find undiscovered skin cancers.

Sophia Haywood, Work Experience Student, UK

2. Optimise your learning time, and learn specific flash cards for specific learning experiences, e.g. if you are about to watch hip replacement surgery, in the spare 10 minutes while waiting for the consultant to scrub up, refresh your mind on the anatomy of the hip.

Note

To use flashcards more efficiently, a specific method can be employed, to maximise your learning potential. The method works by recalling a fact from a flash card; if you recall the fact correctly you put it into the next pile. If you don't then the card goes back into the pile. You move the cards up and down the piles as you get them right or wrong. Your study can then be directed with the appropriate time allocated to learning each group, i.e. the pile that you don't know so well you may choose to revise every day, and the pile you do know well revise every 5 days.

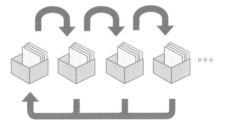

Move a card up to the next pile if you get it right

Move a card down the piles if you get it wrong

6. Look up fundoscopy appearance

Look at a couple of fundoscopy slides, found in clinical examination books, and compare your knowledge to what you find in a patient. Even if there is no abnormality, it's good to practice knowing where the optic disc, macula, etc are.

Guarav Asal, Medical Student, UK

Taking it a step further

1. Test a friend by using clinical pictures as flash cards; can they tell you whether this is macular degeneration or a normal eye?

2. Look at clinical examination books for pictures of the tympanic membrane, and learn these along side the technique of using a otoscope (see Section 4).

---

7. Quiz yourself in theatre

If you are in surgery and you do not have the opportunity to scrub up, or there is no space at the table, take the time to test your knowledge of the surgery.

For example, during a thyroidectomy try to recite everything you know about thyroid diseases. This includes types and prevalence, symptoms, clinical signs, treatment and if possible the examination for it. Once you have exhausted your thoughts look through a clinical handbook for things you have missed. 10 minutes later try and remember them all again reciting them to a partner.

Kayur Patel, Medical Student, UK

Taking it a step further

1. Carry out this task in pairs, with one person trying to recite everything that he or she knows about the disease, and the other checking it in a clinical reference book, then swap over for a different topic.

2. Ask the consultant to talk you through the anatomy that you will be seeing throughout the surgery.

Theme: e-learning resources

Background

Early on in your placements, scout out where you can access a computer and the internet. Hospitals invariably have an education suite for junior doctors, which will more than likely have computers available to students, or even more conveniently have internet access on the wards. With hundreds of medical websites online, varying from tutorials to workshops, to medical games or journals, it really means that even on the quietest day on the wards, there is always something constructive you could do with your time to broaden your understanding and increase your learning of medical matters.

Requirements

A computer with internet access.

8. Websites for information

When I was a foundation year 1 house officer, I found myself getting bored on most surgical nights. As I am not one of those who could sleep their way through the night knowing the bleep might just go off any time, I prefer to stay awake doing something constructive but not too taxing. I would go to www.emedicine.com or www.bmjlearning.com and choose a module to do. It only takes about 10–15 minutes to update myself on a certain topic and at the end of the module, I get a certificate from the website which I could proudly compile into my portfolio as evidence of my learning! By doing just a few modules, I have never failed to learn something on my nights! Not to mention that it is easier at night when most computers are free and you don't get as many calls!

Saw Sian Khoo, Doctor, Malaysia

www.instantanatomy.net for nuggets of anatomy knowledge in brief, simple style that is good for quick learning and revision. Covers whole body in general.

www.wikipedia.org for lots of information on all aspects of medical science. Good for quick look up of information.

Ravinder Pabla, Doctor, UK

9. Websites for revision

Get to a computer with internet access and log on to www.joint-zone.org.uk. It is a website looking at the core knowledge required for those undergraduate rheumatology placements and exams. So no longer will you be wandering the hospital wards for those rheumatology inpatients that don't exist, you will be brushing up on your knowledge, preparing to diagnose that next stiff joint.

Log on to **www.surgical-tutor.org.uk**. It's a great website aimed at those preparing for undergraduate and postgraduate surgical examinations. Great if you are interested in surgery and want to learn more about a specific field, and even better if you just want to brush up on your surgical knowledge and revise. No longer will you be caught out on the surgical ward round during consultant interrogation, and termed for the rest of your placement 'stupid boy!'.

Ashley Simpson, Medical Student, UK

10. Research national guidelines

www.nice.org.uk and **www.sign.ac.uk** for guidelines in management of wide range of conditions with evidence base to justify practice. Easy to search as categorised by topic, speciality and alphabet.

Ravinder Pabla, Doctor, UK

In my recent paediatrics placement the consultants often recommended the junior doctors to check the protocols of certain treatments, for example treatment for a seizing child. Sometimes protocols can differ between Trusts, and hospitals. In a spare 5 minutes check the protocols for the treatment of some of the patients on your ward, or that have been discussed at hand over.

Abigail Cole, Medical Student, UK

Taking it a step further

1. Patient websites are often very good at presenting information in a clear and concise way, and although you may not get an in-depth account of pathology, a brief overview can often be very useful. Try **www.patient.co.uk** and **www.cks.nhs.uk/information_for_patients**.

2. Check out videos of patients with certain diseases to give another perspective on how it can affect their life. Check out **www.childrenfirst.nhs.uk** for the Great Ormond Street Hospital website, which has some useful videos.

3. Enter medical symptoms into **YouTube** to get videos of symptoms and how they can present. An example is croup; this gives some good videos of children with a typical 'barking' cough.

3. Online forums are great places to gain an idea of patients' experiences of certain medical procedures. For example, typing 'ileostomy' into **Google** brings up several forums where the patients' personal experiences of having this procedure is documented, and is a useful tool as a medical student to have some understanding of the day-to-day difficulties/issues faced by these patients.

4. Professional bodies tend to publish their own lists of guidelines – examples include the British Association for Sexual Health and HIV (**www.BASHH.org**) and the Royal College of Obstetricians and Gynaecologists (**www.RCOG.org.uk**).

Cross-references

As stated in the introduction to this section, there is overlap between this section and other sections of the book; you may wish to look explicitly at the following themes for more tips on learning effectively.

For peer practice of physical examination skills	Section 3
For peer practice of practical skills	Section 4
Using and improving peers as a source of feedback	e.g. Tasks 15, 24, 40
Data interpretation – learning from test results, investigations	e.g. Tasks 79 onward, Section 7
Some excellent suggestions related to prescribing and pharmacology	see Section 5

References/further reading

An introduction to concepts of active learning
Spencer JA, Jordan RK (1999). Learner centred approaches in medical education. *BMJ* **318**:1280–3.

Study skills for higher education, for medical education
Cottrell S (2003). *The Study Skills Handbook*. Basingstoke: Palgrave Macmillan.
Cottrell S (2003). *Skills for Success: The personal development planning handbook*. Basingstoke: Palgrave Macmillan.
Buzan T (1995). *Use your Head*. London: BBC.
Evans D, Brown J (2009). *How to Succeed at Medical School: An essential guide to learning*. Oxford: Wiley-Blackwell.

Mnemonics and memory
Brown M (1977). *Memory Matters*. Newon Abbot: David & Charles.
Miller GA (1956). The magical number seven, plus or minus two: Some limits on our capacity for processing information. *Psychol Rev* **63**:81–97.

What kind of learner are you?
For finding that learning style suits you best try filling in the questionnaire at **www.vark-learn.com**.

Section 2
CLINICAL COMMUNICATION

Spend time clerking different patients especially if you are a third year medical student, that's the easiest thing to do.

Ijeoma Akunna, Medical Student, UK

Introduction

Words are, of course, the most powerful drug used by mankind

Rudyard Kipling

This section focuses mainly on clinical communication, which looks at a broad range of areas. It includes history taking, understanding the patient's story, observing communication skills in others and some specific communication situations such as discharge planning. In general, clinical communication is divided into information gathering (history taking), information giving (explaining) and exploring. You will notice that submissions for this book have tended to focus on history taking ('clerking' patients, timed histories, medication histories) and exploring (the patient's story, discharge planning) with very little on explaining. This may reflect the roles of medical students on the wards, but don't forget that developing your skills in explaining is also important to prepare for life as a doctor.

Clinical communication skills are important to be a good doctor. If done right, an order of 75% of diagnoses can be made after taking a history alone. Good communication skills have been shown to have more positive outcomes in terms of patient satisfaction and a wide range of physiological outcomes, including control of hypertension and diabetes. In addition to poorer patient outcomes, poor communication skills make a significant contribution to about 70% of malpractice litigation cases.

This book is clearly not a book on clinical communication skills, but simply a collection of tasks that students and faculty have suggested could be useful to fill 'spare time' on the wards. We would highly recommend reading at least the first chapter (11 pages) of the book by Suzanne Kurtz and her colleagues listed under Further reading – it should be available in your library and makes an easy read.

Your medical school is likely to have its preferred frameworks for thinking about communication. As part of the introduction we give a brief overview of two of the most common frameworks. We present these rather briefly, but you can find more information under Further reading.

Process versus content

Both frameworks rely on the integration of content (the 'what') and process (the 'how'). If taking a focused history from a patient with chest pain, the **content** that you will need to cover includes site of pain, onset, character, radiation, etc., relevant past history, risk factors for cardiovascular disease, medication and so forth. The **process** will reflect how you go about gathering this information (your questioning style and blend of open and closed questions, whether you follow the patient's story or follow your own agenda, your non-verbal communication, the way that you do or do not demonstrate empathy, etc.).

The reason for highlighting this is that it is essential to blend appropriate content with appropriate process, in order to communicate effectively in medicine. Clinical communication skills and medical knowledge are therefore intimately related, and this should be reflected in the way that you go about learning them.

The Calgary–Cambridge guide (Kurtz et al. 1998)

This model separates the consultation into stages:

- Initiating the session
- Gathering information, including both the biomedical perspective (disease) and the patient's perspective (illness), alongside other relevant information
- Physical examination
- Explanation and planning
- Closing the session.

Throughout these stages, there are two ongoing parallel processes in play:

1. Providing structure (through signposting, summarising, etc.)
2. Building a professional relationship (developing rapport, involving the patient, appropriate non-verbal behaviour, etc.).

The patient-centred clinical interview (Stewart 1995)

This model highlights the separate but parallel searches of both the 'disease framework' and the 'illness framework'. The exploration of the biomedical model/disease framework/'doctor's agenda' (to make a diagnosis) is through the traditional history, examination and investigation. The exploration of the illness framework/patient's perspective/'patient's agenda' (for understanding how the disease affects the patient) is through identifying the patient's ideas, expectations and feelings, and the effect of the illness on his or her functioning.

As with the Calgary–Cambridge guide, this model also identifies many of the key skills required: attentive listening, appropriate questioning style, clarification, summarising, rapport building, etc.

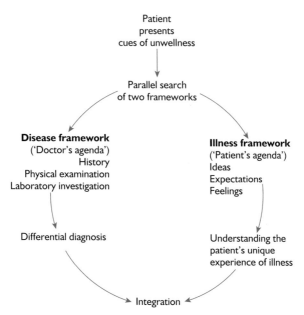

Patient
presents
cues of unwellness

Parallel search
of two frameworks

Disease framework
('Doctor's agenda')
History
Physical examination
Laboratory investigation

Differential diagnosis

Illness framework
('Patient's agenda')
Ideas
Expectations
Feelings

Understanding the
patient's unique
experience of illness

Integration

The patient-centred clinical interview.

Learning clinical communication

As with any skill, learning clinical communication skills requires knowledge, practice (and plenty of it) and feedback (p. 32). The **knowledge** of how to take a focused history from a patient with haemoptysis, for example, requires knowing both the content and the processes required. Your knowledge of the content will be gained from your knowledge of basic science, clinical medicine books and pathology books, and through the experience of watching others. Your knowledge of process will be gained from your communication skills training, communication skills books (and formal models such as the Calgary–Cambridge guide above), and watching both good and less ideal role-models in practice. Of course, abstract knowledge is not enough. Your reading from books needs to be translated into practical knowledge that can be applied in real-life situations, and this translation occurs only through practice and feedback.

   Practice is important, both in simulation ('role-play') and with patients and colleagues. This practice needs to be thoughtful and frequent, and informed by useful **feedback**. The literature shows that medical students around the world are only rarely observed taking histories by staff on the wards, and so your peers will form an important source of feedback (in Tasks 15 & 40 we specifically address how to make this as effective as possible). Remember patients will also be a useful source of feedback: if you have explained your role properly (i.e. as a student, there to learn), they are likely to be keen and willing to help you learn – all you have to do is ask!

What is in this chapter?

This chapter covers four main themes in the submissions. The **patient's story or narrative** features highly in the submissions, and we include some suggestions for advanced practice and interesting reading about this increasingly recognised aspect of clinical communication. We provide some practical suggestions on **preparing** for history taking, including how to construct proformas, feedback forms and how to engage in peer practice. **History taking** features, of course, and includes some innovative ideas for 'histories in a hurry', alongside specialist histories. Finally, there is a great deal to learn from **observing others' communication** and in this theme we cluster some suggestions on how to learn from both the good and the less ideal communication that you will see going on around you.

Omissions from this chapter

As mentioned above, this book is constructed from submissions by students, staff and others. These submissions are fantastic, and we are sure that you will find them invaluable; we have, however, noticed some areas that are not extensively covered in the submissions, including written communication, telephone communication, and communication between different professionals, whether of the same profession or between different professions, including handovers and referrals. There are no submissions relating to chronic care histories, nutritional histories, or histories exploring drug and alcohol use. We hope that you find the submissions that we have included here stimulating, but please do not be limited by them, and if you find other communication skills 'things to do' in your spare moments, why not consider submitting them to **www.101things.org**.

Summary
Clinical communication skills are essential for the practice of medicine. You will need to attend to both content and process, and should include both the biomedical perspective and the patient's perspective. As with any skill, developing good clinical communication skills will take many years of deliberate and thoughtful practice, starting with your first day on the wards.

Theme: narrative – the patient's story

Background

History taking involves more than just gathering facts in order to make a diagnosis. It is important to gain an understanding of the patient's story – his or her narrative. From the most pragmatic view, exploring the patient's narrative will help you to build rapport, resulting in a range of positive outcomes, in terms of both patient satisfaction and biomedical outcomes. It will also help you to understand the impact that patients' symptoms have on their lives, which will enable you to plan and prioritise your management in order to improve the quality of **this** patient's life. Within a medical culture which can sometimes dehumanise patients ('the hysterectomy in bed 5'), the patient's story also allows you to see the person beyond and before the diagnosis. Advanced narrative approaches (see 'Taking it a step further') can encourage you to see yourself as a person, as a human affected by the humans around you.

For many, putting the 'person' before the science will be central to how they choose to practise medicine throughout their professional lives – it comes with some emotional cost, but also brings huge satisfaction. Medical school is a perfect time to start, as shown by the range of suggestions submitted.

Requirements

A patient (or relative), who is willing to talk.

---

11. Patient story

Why restrict yourself to task-oriented patient contact?

Patients have so much more to offer! A 10–30 minute visit 'just for a chat' to see how patients are feeling, without bombarding them with history-taking, etc. can often be far more educational than any other type of visit. I've found that a quick visit post ward round can make the patient feel that you're interested in them as a whole, and you get a valuable glimpse of medicine from 'the other side of the bed'. Often, they will confide in you during this time, telling you their true concerns – fears that perhaps they were too afraid to mention on the hurried ward round when a gaggle of medics are gawping down at them! The things that trouble them most may be simple for a medical student to fix, and will improve their experience of being a patient. I would recommend asking 'If I had a magic wand right now, what could I do for you?'. You may be surprised by the answer you get, as what's important to us as clinicians is often of secondary importance to the patient.

I've used this approach since my first day on firms, and cannot stress how helpful it's been in the holistic learning process!

In addition, for those wishing to impress their consultant, nothing works better than a patient greeting a student, by name, with a broad grin, enthusing about how helpful they've been

Emma Court, Medical Student, UK

If there isn't much going on, the doctors are busy, and patients have all been clerked or are tired, just go and chat to those patients who are awake, or those who haven't had a visitor for a while. Find out about them, how they are feeling about being in hospital, offer to pop to the shop for them or make them a cuppa. When they are feeling more 'with it', they are usually more than happy to give you an hour or two of their day so that you can take a full history and perform multiple systems examinations.

Not only do you get to practise your skills, you also get invaluable information about how patients feel about being 'inside', and about people's health beliefs.

Joanne Evans, Medical Student, UK

The patient that wanted to talk for ages on the ward round ... go back and talk to him/her, they might have something interesting to say and, if not, you made their day happier and worked on your communication skills. Plus the next time they need blood taking or a cannula in, they'll remember you and let you do it.

Kathryn Rhodes, Medical Student, UK

I'm only a first year medical student but have recently read a book on doctor communication. It became apparent that in a hospital environment the doctor can often express his own agenda more than that of the patient. In my time I spent on the wards before medical school I realised that you can learn fascinating things about patients that you would never have guessed by looking at them.

Therefore what harm is there if you have a few minutes free, here and there, to talk to a patient in a non-medical sense, and just query about their past and feelings, etc.

This may sound a bit like a volunteer's job, but in a sense it should greatly improve that doctor–patient relationship. The patient then feels the doctor is genuinely interested in them, rather than trying to cure them and get them out ASAP to clear up a bed!

There's psychology studies to show that a good and positive mood improves recovery time, so by doing this, potentially you will make the patient feel better in themselves!

Andrew Smith, Medical Student, UK

Patients get bored on the ward too.

Go and chat to one of the patients on the ward with no particular agenda apart from being an interested human being. Allow the patient to take the conversation where they want to go. Be prepared to share something about yourself while maintaining comfortable and appropriate boundaries.

You'll probably come away feeling a bit more energised and positive.

You'll probably find out things that help put that patient's illness in context and may offer insights into their care.

You might come away feeling less bored but with a lower mood.

Consultations influence our mood and you need to be able to recognise this. Take a look at some of the models of the consultation at a later time.

Andy Wearn, Clinical Senior Lecturer, New Zealand

Taking it a step further

It is not only the patient who is affected by ill health and the healthcare system; the effect on relatives can also be profound, and often goes unnoticed.

12. Learning from relatives

Make contact with a partner/relative of a patient and ask about his/her experiences with healthcare professionals. Ask about doctors' professional behaviour, his/her provision of information and educational activities. Ask for two examples that helped the relative in the whole process of supporting the patient and ask for two examples that frustrated him/her. Benefit from these examples by reflecting on your own professional behaviour.

Of course you can translate this idea to other personal talks. Need examples? Talk to patients, other healthcare professionals and ask for examples of good and frustrating doctor practices, if you desire focus on a certain aspect of doctor's professional behaviour.

Jolien van den Houten, Occupational Therapist, The Netherlands

13. Parallel charts

Every day you will write down the patient history and examination in the prescribed format (PC – presenting complaint, HPC – history of presenting complaint, PMH – past medical history, SH – social history, etc.). Sometimes you will write this in the hospital notes, at other times you will write it on paper to carry around with you, ensuring that it is anonymous. This standardised format will be with you for the rest of your professional life and will direct your thinking and your clinical reasoning. However, there will be things that arise that do not fit into the standard, prescribed format. Perhaps these are things that patients say about their family, their home or their past history. Perhaps there are things about how the patient makes you feel, that they remind you of someone that you are close to, or that you dislike, or perhaps that you feel hopeful or helpless for them. Writing these things down, in a parallel set of notes ('parallel chart'), will capture these thoughts and feelings, when they might otherwise have been lost in the process of writing. As a result you may find your learning extending past the biomedical model of medicine. Consider getting a group of like-minded students together where you can share these 'parallel charts'.

'... the goals are to enable them [the students] to recognise more fully what their patients endure and examine explicitly their own journeys through medicine. This textual work is a practical and, I believe, essential part of medical training, designed to increase the students' capacity for effective clinical work.'

Concept and quotation from Charon (2006)
Suggestion from Shmuel Reis, Senior Faculty, Israel

Theme: preparation

Background

History taking isn't easy to learn. When starting out you will struggle to balance the different parts of history taking: weighing up the information that you are gathering and what it might mean (and so where they should explore next) against building rapport and exploring the patient's perspective. To make things even more frustrating, experts can generally do it all very quickly and often unconsciously, making it look far simpler than it is.

There is a separate and important skill of documentation. Most clinicians will write down the history as they talk to the patient, but a few will just write down things that they will find difficult to remember, and write the full notes after the consultation. Writing while listening, talking and maintaining rapport is a skill in its own right. Some of these suggestions may help you develop this skill.

Within this theme there are a couple of suggestions in which to prepare for this complex skill set. None of these suggestions replaces practice with patients, but they will help prepare and help you continuously improve.

Requirements

Some spare time, some paper, possibly a clinical communication skills book and a decent clinical medicine and/or clinical surgery book are all that are required.

14. History proforma

Write out headings if you are waiting to see a patient. Get a blank piece of paper and write out headings such as 'presenting complaint', 'history of presenting complaint', etc. If you have some indication of the patient's reason for being in hospital, think of questions to ask them. Use this time also to gather demographic information about them (e.g. DOB, date of admission, etc.). This is also a good time to try to find their drug chart and make a note of all their medications. Type up the headings you use and keep copies ready (with spaces to write); this should mean you don't have to look for paper, don't waste valuable history sheets and don't forget important parts of the history.

Donna Arya, Medical Student, UK

Notes

1. This can be a useful tool for reminding you of the different areas of the history to explore. Do not feel that you need to explore them in the order on your piece of paper; follow the patient's story, writing your notes in the correct place on your proforma as you go along.

2. Name, age and occupation traditionally come at the top of the patient notes and at the start of the case presentation. You do not, however, need to start asking the history with these questions – a patient who is touchy about his or her age, or who has just lost a job may find these questions intrusive, especially before you have built any rapport with him or her. Experiment by putting these questions later in the history taking.

---

15. Constructing a feedback form

By far the most frequent person to watch you communicating with patients and give you feedback will be another student. This has some advantages over a senior doctor, particularly as a colleague tends to be less intimidating, but also has some disadvantages – their knowledge of appropriate content and process might be poorer, and they may not be as skilled in giving feedback as an experienced teacher. They may also be reluctant to give you feedback on areas where you need to improve. Using a suitable proforma can help guide the feedback and so improve its usefulness and effectiveness.

Construct a clinical communication feedback form, either alone or in collaboration with some other students. Make one generic form based on the formal model of clinical communication used at your school (perhaps Calgary–Cambridge guide, which even has two suggested feedback forms in its appendix). Use this form to structure your observations of others and feedback on their clinical communication and ask them to use it when they watch you. It will help them provide more detailed feedback, and also to notice the things that you do well, alongside the things that you could or should change.

Dason Evans, Doctor and Author

Taking it a step further

1. You can make these forms as wide or as closed as you like. For example, you might work with others and some clinical medicine textbooks to produce a feedback form for a certain task, such as taking a history of chest pain or explaining type 2 diabetes. These forms could include both content and process items, to allow you to give feedback on both when seeing a relevant patient. This isn't a bad method for revising clinical medicine either!

2. You might produce some specific feedback forms for other things – breaking bad news, discharge planning, handover between healthcare professionals. You will find that these will help you to critique the communication that you see occurring around you, and learn from other people's approaches (Task 20).

Note: there is no one way of communicating and one doctor may take a totally different approach to another with the same task for the same patient. One doctor is likely to take different approaches for different patients, so use these proformas for feedback, but not to memorise some sort of ultimate 'right way'.

---

16. Peer practice

I found that at my time as a third year at district general hospitals not always, but often, the junior doctors had too much to do and the seniors were busy elsewhere. There were times that, between all of us, all the patients on the wards had been clerked, no more bloods and cannulas needed doing. Still wanting to make the most of our time, however, a colleague and myself would go down to the canteen, get a cup of coffee and sit in the quietest corner, either one of us pretending to be a patient (chest pain, abdo pain, haematemesis, etc.), bearing in mind a particular condition, and the other student took a history. That student then presented the history back and we went on to talk about all the conditions that present in that manner (using the Oxford Handbook of Clinical Medicine and a differential diagnosis book of course for reference).

Devangi Thakkar, Medical Student, UK

Theme: history taking

Background

The medical history ('clerking') is the foundation of the entire consultation. At its most basic it is about three things: understanding the patient, building a therapeutic relationship, and building/testing a hypothesis for diagnosis and treatment. None of these three aspects is easy – and for the rest of your professional life you will get it right some of the time, and other times leave a consultation thinking about what you could have done differently. One thing is clear: although practice might not make perfect, thoughtful practice and feedback do result in improvement – clerking patients should be the bread and butter of a medical student's life on the wards.

Requirements

You will need a willing patient, of course, and remember that one patient may be willing and suitable for various history-taking tasks. The bored patient with diabetes who has been admitted with a myocardial infarction may be happy to help you learn to take a history of chest pain, or even a diabetic history, medication history, nutrition history, etc., in addition to a full history during their inpatient stay.

As with any skill, being observed by a student colleague or clinician will help you to receive constructive feedback, and understand where you can make improvements. You might improve the quality of this feedback by using a feedback proforma (Task 15).

17. Clerking patients

There should be trained staff around — ask if there are any interesting patients (particularly under your consultant). Go and clerk them! Obtain a history and examine them (the latter might not always be appropriate but general observations are always very useful). You should take as much time as you have spare. Then you can present the case to the consultant on the ward round the next day/in surgery or to someone in your team. There may be something extra you have obtained from the history that was not previously recognised — you can add this in the notes. This hones your history-taking skills to the particular complaint and provides you with a patient's face and background on which you can link with your reading on the topic later.

Laura Geddes, Medical Student, UK

Timed histories

OSCE (Objective Structured Clinical Exams) preparation features heavily in the submissions for this book, particularly at exam time. Remember, however, that, if you can take a rapid, focused and appropriate history of chest pain in 5 minutes, or explain the diagnosis and management of type 2 diabetes effectively in 10 minutes, these skills will serve you well throughout your career, as well as in OSCEs.

Practising history taking and explaining procedures to patients, with a student colleague acting as an examiner can be hugely helpful. Please remember to ask nursing staff before approaching patients.

Patients are the best people to give you feedback on how they feel about your communication skills. Tell them that you want them to be as open as possible and that you will not take offence.

Also nurse specialists are experts in their field and can give you great feedback. When asking for feedback, remember to tell them it will only take about 10 minutes. We are supposed to be able to do these OSCE stations in 6 minutes and that gives them a few minutes to give you feedback.

Canh Van On, Medical Student, UK

See also
Task 27.

While I'm here – histories in a hurry

There will be opportunities to take histories when involved with other activities with patients; these 'snatched moments' can be incredibly powerful for learning.

When taking blood from patients, utilise the time with the patient well — take a history while preparing the bottles, and then assess why each sample is being taken and its relevance to the case. This way, history-taking, thought process and phlebotomy skills are all being exercised at the same time. Plus, the houseman will be thankful for it! Just watch out for needlestick injuries.

Paul Cacciottolo, Medical Student, Malta

Go along during meal times and ask the nurses if there are any patients that require help with feeding. Whether it is actively feeding the patient or just sitting with them to give them company and encouragement, it's a great feeling to be actually doing something worthwhile, and you'll probably get the patient's story too.

Laura Cohen, Medical Student, UK

18. Discharge planning

Talking about discharge planning and about activities of daily living (ADLs) such as whether the patient can manage to cook, dress, clean, climb stairs, etc. in the house is an important skill. It's a good way to gauge how a patient is feeling about going home and good practice for students. It's also a nice way to continue caring for the patient until they go home, as the student may have clerked the patient earlier regarding their admission.

Sabrina Talukdar, Medical Student, UK

Taking it a step further

Sit down with your colleagues and brainstorm on other places where you might take a history – examples might include the ECG department, the radiology department, day case surgery – the list you will come up with will be a long one.

19. Focused histories

Brainstorm also to come up with a list of different focused histories that you should be familiar and competent with. These might include histories relating to a range of presenting symptoms (diarrhoea, chest pain, nose-bleeds etc ...) and might also include more specialist histories such as discharge planning and medication history, above, nutritional history, detailed family history of genetic disease, etc. Again, you will form a long list of skills to learn and practise.

Strangely, there were no submissions for this book that covered chronic disease histories (e.g. a patient transferring to a neurologist with a long history of debilitating multiple sclerosis, or a patient joining a new general practice with a long history of complicated diabetes). These histories are quite different in content and approach when compared to an acute event history. Why not investigate the differences, and even submit an idea to share with others – **www.101things.org**.

See also

Section 5 includes some tasks around taking a medication history (Task 59).

Theme: observing communication

Background

You will spend a great deal of your time during clinical attachments watching others communicate – whether on ward rounds, clinics, anaesthetic rooms, between doctors and patients or between different members of the healthcare team, it is going on all the time. Often students are so immersed in it that they don't even notice the opportunity for learning around them.

Over the years you will see every possible form of communication occurring around you. You will see some fantastic role models and can learn a great deal from them. You will see plenty of less optimal communication, which will also provide excellent opportunities for reflection and learning. The secret is to train yourself to become aware of what is happening around you.

Indeed, it is not unusual to sit in outpatient clinics or general practice and become a little bored, especially in subspecialty clinics where the management of patients may be so advanced, or so repetitive, that you lose interest. In these situations, rather than day dream or try to subtly thumb through a pocket textbook, spend some time looking at the doctor–patient interaction – within this theme you will find some suggestions on how to do this effectively.

Requirements

Any communication occurring around you. Your eyes and your ears.

---

20. Learning from the great communicators, learning from the others

Over the years you will see a huge range of communication skills on display. Some will be ones that you want to adopt; others will be approaches that you decide you would like to avoid.

I find that one learns the most from watching the consultants and other doctors – making mistakes!

For instance one morning, the consultant we were assigned to showed us a little 74-year-old lady with lung cancer. He started discussing the diagnosis quietly with us, and mentioned cancer. Before his words had time to sink in, the patient's eyes opened wide in shock: 'Am I going to die?', she asked.

The consultant realised his mistake – he had discussed the patient's condition in front of her, but not with her. He had wrongly assumed that the patient was hard of hearing. Not only did we all learn a valuable lesson on bedside manners, we also got to see the consultant try to salvage the situation.

Rachelle Asciak, Medical Student, Malta

Keep a couple of pages in a notebook and jot down useful terms or phrases and effective approaches to communicating about sensitive topics; decide how you might adapt these to your own style.

Dason Evans, Doctor and Author

Taking it a step further

1. Use the feedback form that you created above (Task 15) to structure your observations of other people's communication skills, and ask them to use it when critiquing you. You can even use the same form to analyse communication skills that you see on TV medical soaps! Clearly, any observation of senior or other qualified staff should be handled discretely.

2. Keep a list of specific communication skills challenges in your portfolio, and keep adding to it as you come across more (working with interpreters is a good example). Work out how you are going to address these challenges. Some students even start study groups specifically for clinical communication development.

3. In addition to understanding **language** that varies between different members of a multidisciplinary team, a good communicator will pick up on **cues** during an interaction. These are verbal or non-verbal hints that suggest an underlying emotion in need of clarification. If we pick these up, especially during consultations with patients, we would have happier patients and shorter clinics.

A recent study by Levinson (2000) suggested that GP consultations that were **cue** based were on average 15% shorter than those in which **cues** were more frequently missed. See if you can spot cues during any interaction with a patient when either you or someone else is carrying out a consultation. The better you become at spotting them, the shorter your clinic appointments and happier your patients will be.

Sheetal Patel, Economist, UK

21. Breaking bad news

Shadow your senior medical staff and ask to sit in and watch how bad news/death is broken to patients or their relatives. Then role-play with your peers, although it is quite different from reality, practice certainly improves you ability to break bad news.

Su Ping Ho, Medical Student, UK

Breaking bad news is something that we all dread; yet we all have to learn the skill. If someone is going to perform this, ask kindly if you can attend. Even though you are part of the medical team, stand quietly at the back and just observe. There is a lot to learn: the way to break bad news, how body language can help and how you can deal with patients' reactions. Last, but not least by any means, of the moral and ethical questions and dilemmas that can arise.

Laura Geddes, Medical Student, UK

Notes

1. There are some formal models for breaking bad news, such as the six-step approach (Baile et al. 2000). Have a look at the model that your school advocates. How well does it reflect practice? What is the reasoning behind the model and how will it affect your practice?

2. Many clinicians will be reluctant to have a student present when they are breaking bad news. They are more likely to allow you in if they know you and that you are keen to learn. You may suggest that you will 'stand quietly at the back and just observe'. It sometimes may not be appropriate for a student to be present in these situations, so you should be keen but not pushy.

3. Role-playing sensitive topics, such as breaking bad news, can bring back painful memories for some students; look at Task 40 and think about how you might adapt this task for clinical communication skills role-plays.

See also

The section 'Being curious' includes tasks related to understanding communication in other professions including nursing handover (Task 67). This can be extended to any of the tasks involving other professions – see, for example, (Task 44 to 46).

22. Communicating to children

Children require a specialised form of communication. In order for you to engage with them you often have to play and interact with them first. You will also learn that your ability to communicate with them will vary according to the age of the patient, their familiarity with you and many other factors beyond your understanding or control! A useful person to learn from is the play specialist.

When you are doing your paediatrics placement try to spend some time with the play therapist. Seeing how they explain procedures to children and demonstrate these procedures by involving the child in play will be valuable experience when you have to go and take blood, insert a Venflon or perform other such procedures on a child.

Alison Bradley, Medical Student, UK

Taking it a step further

Keep a log of all your interactions with children and list those things that you did well and those that could be improved and see if there is any progress with time.

Sangita Patel, Teacher, UK

23. Communication challenges

Identify those patients with special communication needs on the ward and brainstorm what additional precautions you would use to improve your communication. Examples of those with challenging communication needs include patients with poor hearing, no or little English, inability to speak (i.e. tracheostomy patients) and those with learning needs. Afterwards you could try taking a medical history from each of these patients and see if your techniques were effective.

Sheetal Patel, Economist, UK

References/further reading

Overview of learning clinical communication skills
Evans DE, Brown J (2009). Learning clinical communication skills. In: *How to Succeed at Medical School: An essential guide to learning*. Oxford: Blackwells/BMJ Books.

The Calgary–Cambridge approach
Kurtz SM, Silverman J, Draper J (1998). *Teaching and Learning Communication Skills in Medicine*. Abingdon, Oxon: Radcliffe Medical Press.
Kurtz S, Silverman J, Benson J, Draper J (2003). Marrying content and process in clinical method teaching: Enhancing the Calgary–Cambridge guides. *Acad Med* **78**:802–9.

The patient-centred clinical interview

Baile WF, Buckman R, Lenzi R, Glober G, Beale, EA, Kudelka AP (2000). SPIKES – A six-step protocol for delivering bad news: application to the patient with cancer. *Oncologist* **5**:302–11.

Stewart M (1995) *Patient-centered Medicine: Transforming the clinical method*. Thousand Oaks, CA: Sage.

Stewart M, Roter D (1989). *Communicating with Medical Patients*. Thousand Oaks, CA: Sage.

Parallel Charts

Charon R (2006). *Narrative Medicine: Honoring the stories of illness*. New York: Oxford University Press: Chapter 8.

Patient Cues

Levinson W (2000). Improving communication with patients. *Hosp Pract* (Minneap). Apr 15;**35**(4):113–4, 117–20; discussion 120, 123.

Section 3
PHYSICAL EXAMINATION

He who studies medicine without books sails an uncharted sea, but he who studies medicine without patients does not go to sea at all.

William Osler (1849–1919)

Introduction

Why clinical skills are important

Clinical skills (including communication skills, physical examination skills and practical procedures) form the core skills that define the medical profession. Your eyes, hands and ears will form the most important diagnostic tools in your armoury for the rest of your life. This section principally covers physical examination skills, and there are other sections on practical skills and clinical communication; however, this introduction is relevant to all three aspects,

Imagine the skill of examining a pregnant woman close to the time of delivery. By looking at her as she walks in you can make many spot diagnoses; you can exclude joint problems (spine and pelvis, for example) that are common in later pregnancy. By looking at the woman's skin and eyes as she walks closer, you can assess whether you think she might be significantly anaemic, and exclude jaundice and excoriations that might be related to liver problems in pregnancy. Her hands, pulse, ankles and blood pressure will tell you a great deal about her current and past health, and help you exclude life-threatening pre-eclampsia. Examining her abdomen will help you identify if this pregnancy is high risk (small or large baby, little or excess amniotic fluid, scars representing previous uterine surgery, transverse or oblique lie representing risk of cord prolapse), or if all is normal. The way that you examine this woman, and the explanation that you give while you examine her, will help you build a rapport with her, and help her become involved, a true partner in her care.

Good clinical skills are, therefore, crucial to patient care. In this book we have separated out physical examination skills, practical skills and communication skills into different sections. This separation is artificial, but convenient for the purpose of this book.

How to learn clinical skills

It is worthwhile remembering that to learn any skill you need to know how to perform it, you need to practise and practise plenty, and you need to receive and act on constructive feedback (the Evans–Brown model 2009).

According to the Michels' Framework (2012) the knowledge of how to perform a skill contains more than just the **steps** involved; it also includes the **basic science** behind

101 Things to Do with Spare Moments on the Ward, First Edition. Dason E Evans, Nakul Gamanlal Patel. © 2012 Dason E Evans and Nakul Gamanlal Patel. Published 2012 by Blackwell Publishing Ltd.

the steps (anatomy, physiology, etc.) so that you understand what you are doing and can adapt in different situations, and finally it includes **clinical reasoning**, both what the procedure might tell you and under what circumstances it might be useful.

Medical students tend to have a proven track record in learning knowledge, but learning a skill is fundamentally different from learning knowledge, so we would strongly encourage you to spend some time thinking about the best way of learning a given skill.

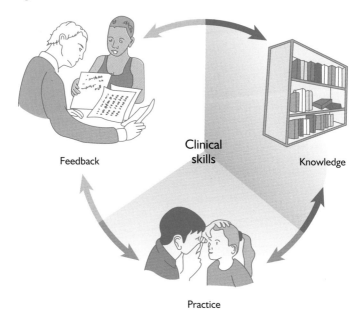

Feedback   Clinical   Knowledge
                  skills

Practice

There is a chapter on the subject in Evans and Brown (2009) (see reference at the end of the chapter).

A great deal of deliberate, thoughtful practice is required to develop expertise (of the order of 10 000 hours, much less to become 'good enough') and, in general, you should aim to practise in within a realistic context (i.e. preferably with real, consenting patients, without having looked at the notes first). Also remember the importance of asking for feedback.

You will find one particular challenge on the wards: for most skills there is no one right way, and clinicians have various different approaches. This is not surprising; we know that many sportsmen and musicians have different approaches to performing their skill, within a generally accepted norm. The surprising thing is that most of these clinicians, although they acknowledge that their colleagues may have different approaches, will try to convince you that their particular approach is the right and indeed the 'only' one. One of your jobs on the wards is to explore different approaches that you are shown or that you read about and start to develop your own style. Clearly this style needs to be within the wide confines of 'normal' practice, so sample widely from clinicians and books and a great deal of practice to gain a consensus of the 'right' approach for you and for a given patient.

Exams on exams
Clinical skills should be learnt to ensure that you can provide excellent patient care as a doctor. Needless to say many students end up focusing on learning for assessments (OSCEs perhaps), and this is reflected in a cluster of suggestions within this section. Remember that around 90% of your time spent practising should be aimed at developing excellent skills for patient care, and perhaps 10% of your time spent fine-tuning your OSCE techniques.

Patient consent and dignity
Clearly ethical behaviour is paramount, and part of this is ensuring that patients have given you consent to examine them, and that you treat them professionally and appropriately; you may wish to read the introduction of this book again for a reminder of some of the issues.

Theme: peer practice for physical examination

Background

There is a lot to think about when examining a patient:

- What is the next 'step' to perform?
- How do I perform that step (where will I put my hands, how best should I instruct the patient, etc.)?
- Am I performing this step right?
- What did the findings from the last step tell me?
- How does this fit in with my other findings so far?
- How can I put this together to present my key findings at the end?
- How will I avoid forgetting my findings as I proceed?
- How am I managing the rapport with the patient?

Many students find it challenging to keep all this in their head at once, which can result in one of two inappropriate behaviours. The first is the student who thinks about nothing other than the steps ('First I do this, then I do this, then I do this'), and misses out on self-critique, learning clinical reasoning and building rapport. These step-driven students learn a ritualised performance without ever understanding the rationale of what they are doing, and they may well become dangerous if allowed to graduate. The second common student reaction to the complexity of examining patients is to hide or put off the challenge until another day. 'Mañana' can and does stretch to months and even years. Because it takes 10 000 hours of deliberate, thoughtful practice to develop expertise, these procrastinating students will run into trouble.

Practising with a colleague allows you to develop some degree of fluency before practising with patients. Many students feel more comfortable stopping and saying 'Hang on, what comes next?' to a colleague than to a patient! Of course, you cannot learn clinical reasoning when examining a colleague, but it's a good start to build up your confidence to examine patients. This is reflected in the number of peer physical examination submissions for this book.

Requirements

A willing colleague, of course, and a suitable environment (see Task 40) with appropriate infection control equipment (sink or alcohol hand rub, paper covers for couch, etc.) are essential. We would recommend having a second colleague there, too, to watch carefully and give feedback; it is hard to be aware of everything that you are doing or having done to you. That third set of eyes may see things that you or your colleague may otherwise miss.

---

24. Peer practice, clinical skills

Practise examination technique, e.g. gait, arms, legs, spine (GALS). Practise on the other person learning the technique. This is a chance to make sure you know the normal movements 100% correctly before having to identify the abnormal with patients.
Of course, the same thing can be done for chest/respiratory, cardiovascular, etc.

Eimeae O'Connor, Medical Student

Just go in an examination room, pick a type of examination, e.g. to examine the shoulder joint or to carry out a respiratory examination... and examine each other. This revisits examination skills and helps to remember exam technique for OSCEs.

Asma Fazlanie, Medical Student, UK

On the wards there's often a doctors' room or office or somewhere where students can go and this is where a lot of time wasting and hanging around occurs. Instead use the spare 5 minutes in between teaching and ward rounds to practise examination techniques. At King's there are exams with 6-minute stations where we have to demonstrate an abdominal exam, or a cardiovascular or respiratory or neurological exam.

If within the spare 5 minutes students were to practise these techniques, it would not only benefit them for the exams but also enable them to be more confident when examining in front of their firm and consultant, and their confidence will be recognised by the patient whose mind will be put at ease. The only equipment that's necessary depends on the examination that you will be practising, so a stethoscope for cardiovascular and respiratory exams and perhaps a tendon hammer for neurological exams, but the examination technique can still be practised without the equipment.

I wish someone had suggested this to me, as revising for the OSCEs wouldn't have felt like such a daunting task with so many examinations to memorise!

May Abboudi, Medical Student, UK

If the ward is ridiculously quiet, try getting a small group together and going into the day room or another room where you won't be shouted at by the nurses for clogging up the corridors, and have a go at practising some examinations together. Neurological is a good one because there's normally reflex hammers and small pin prick needles hanging around a lot of the time. This is particularly good when it gets to exam time and you need to revise but are expected to come in!

Nazia Hossain, Medical Student, UK

25. Practise presenting

Practise presenting patients you've clerked to your peers to improve your fluency and skill in doing this.

Ruth Bird, Medical Student, UK

In the section on practical skills we present some relevant themes and tasks, including:

- Ground rules for peer practice (Task 40)
- Infection control (Tasks 47 and 48).

Taking it a step further

It is not just physical examination that is daunting; putting your findings together and presenting the key features to a consultant ('case presentation') can be intimidating too. Spend some time listening to case presentations on the wards, and practising with your colleagues; see if you can find out the unwritten rules of case presentation – it will serve you very well in the future.

Theme: examining patients – systems examinations

Background

Clinical skills are learnt with patients. Books, lectures, simulation, peer practice and visualisation are all useful techniques for preparing to practise with patients, but in no way replace the huge number of patients whom you will need to examine to learn to recognise pathology from normal variations.

---

26. Examine another patient

If you have spare moments, just go and see another patient, take a history, do a physical examination, write the notes. If you're ever caught sitting waiting – you're out of here!

Shmuel Reis, Head of Medical Education, Haifa, Israel

Practising clinical and communication skills with patients is seen as the bread and butter of clinical training. For many of your clinical supervisors, this is **the** central activity that you should be engaged in on the wards.

If you are new to the wards, it would be worth reviewing the advice about informed consent and the ethical approach to learning with patients. Ensure that all patients know that you are asking to practise for your learning, not their care, and, rest assured, the vast majority of patients will be delighted to help you learn to become a doctor.

Consent to let you practise is a gift from patients; always ensure that they know how grateful you are, both by the things that you say and by the way that you behave toward them.

Requirements

You'll need a willing patient, of course. Have a think about the environment, particularly whether privacy is required, or perhaps a chaperone, and what equipment (including alcohol hand gel) you will need. As with peer physical examination, attention to infection control is essential.

If practising for OSCEs, you might wish to ask someone to time you, so that you become used to what a 5-minute, 10-minute (or in some schools 7-minute) time limit feels like.

Remember, even when practising for OSCEs that the aim is to become an excellent doctor who happens to pass exams along the way, not an excellent exam performer.

27. Practising for OSCEs

Ask a friendly house officer or SHO for a good patient for history and examination. Head off to the patient. One student is the student, while the other student takes on the role of the examiner, and notes and grades the student's performance. The history/examination is timed according to local exam practices (e.g. OSCEs) and, once that time is up, the students discuss what happened.

All findings are to be correlated in the patient's file to ensure accuracy.

Easy to do on the ward and productive on multiple levels.

Paul Cacciottolo, Medical Student, Malta

When bored and in need of some motivation as to why you entered medical school in the first place, go find an SpR or SHO whom you know and ask them to send you to a patient whom they know. Go take a 10-min history (timed by another student) and then ideally ask the SpR or SHO if they will look at you examine that same patient (10 min). Ask them then to ask you questions regarding that presentation.

This often adds a little needed stress (of a mock exam) and keeps the student aware of their abilities and knowledge.

Katharine Elliott, Medical Student, UK

We all have OSCE examinations at the end of the year but at this point our fellow students are equally as stressed and so it can be difficult to find willing volunteers to practise on. A good tip would be to use all those spare 10 minutes and half hours to do your OSCE revision throughout the year.

Identify patients on ward rounds with good clinical signs or ask the FY1 doctor on the ward if any of their patients have good clinical signs. Pair up with a friend; one acts as examiner and one as the student at an OSCE station. Gain consent from the patient and perform one examination. For example, if you find a patient with a heart murmur, perform a full cardiovascular examination on them. The neurology ward is similarly good for practising neurology examination. Afterwards report your findings to your friend who is acting as examiner and then talk through what you missed and how you could improve.

This way you improve your skills and confidence in examination and in reporting findings so that the OSCE exam will not be as daunting. Also by doing short specific examinations the patient is less likely to become bored or tired than if you were fumbling your way through an entire top-to-toe examination for the purposes only of OSCE practice.

Alison Bradley, Medical Student, UK

28. Examining patients for competence

One of the most important aspects of a cardiovascular exam is to describe the heart sounds. In my third year I learnt about the different types of heart murmurs from an SHO, and he told us you need to recognise each one separately. One excellent way to utilise time would be to learn the theory about murmurs, and then go to the cardiology ward and ask any of the doctors to identify patients with murmurs.

Once these patients have been identified, you ask for their consent to be examined. But when you do the examination, ensure you don't know the diagnosis. Listen to the heart sounds first then check if you got it correct or not. If the diagnosis is different then go and listen to the heart sound again. By doing this it will enable the student to appreciate the subtle differences in sound that are present between different murmurs. It will also help improve their overall cardiovascular examination skills, communication skills and give them an opportunity to take more histories.

I believe this is important because a lot of students are not placed on cardiology wards and hence they don't get an opportunity. Also the hearts sounds that are available to listen to on the internet have a poor sound quality.

Bhavin Rawal, Medical Student, UK

Notes

1. A simple adaptation of Bhavin's suggestion would be to conduct a full cardiovascular examination on the patient, trying to guess which valvular lesions might be present **before** even listening to the heart sounds. This deductive reasoning (thinking about diagnosis from the first moment of examination) is an essential part of learning clinical skills.

2. The point that you should avoid looking at the notes until you have made a commitment about the diagnosis is important for learning, as is the point that, if you get it wrong, go back to the patient and try again! If you have asked the patient for consent appropriately, explaining that this is for your learning, then they are likely to be very pleased for you to have another go.

3. Don't forget that the cardiology ward is not the only place to find patients with murmurs (see below).

Don't be restricted to the 'right patients'

Many submissions highlighted that a patient doesn't need to be a 'cardiovascular patient' for you to practise a cardiovascular examination with him or her.

Practise your clinical skills! Go introduce yourself to random patients and ask if they mind if you perform a clinical examination on them or take a history. There's no need for them to be known to you — in fact, it's better if they're not because then you'll have to work out what their diagnosis is. Most patients are happy to let you talk to and examine them; some might even be willing to let you practise your venepuncture skills or other more invasive skills.

Simon Stallworthy, Medical Student, UK

Perform a neurological examination of the upper and lower limbs on any patient (provided the patient is willing and is able to follow commands, of course!). Allow the SHO/registrar to correct your mistakes.

Wei Yang Low, Medical Student, UK

29. Finding patients with signs in other places

Often students reflect on the shortage of 'neurology patients' — remember that you will find plenty of patients with neurology signs in the elderly care wards, rehab wards and even patients with diabetes. For cardiovascular examination an antenatal ward or clinic can prove fruitful: many pregnant women develop ejection systolic murmurs. How might you be able to tell if it is an innocent flow murmur or a potentially life-threatening stenotic aortic valve? Similarly you will find that many elderly patients admitted for other reasons have developed an ejection systolic murmur from aortic sclerosis. Would you be able to tell the difference between this and aortic stenosis? Patients attending for cardiac surgery often have fantastic signs. Is there a pre-clerking clinic you could attend? Remember that a patient with poor coronary blood flow is likely to have poor peripheral blood flow as well … .

Why not produce a list of unexpected places where you can find patients to perform system examinations.

See also
See Section 4 (for practical procedures).

Don't be restricted to 'your' wards: see Sections 6 and 8 for more examples of hidden learning environments. If you have a portfolio, fill the gaps that you have identified by going in search of appropriate patients.

Theme: examining patients – holistic assessments

Background

Much of the **teaching** of clinical skills is based around examining one system or another. However, in medical practice you will often be required to think across systems, to pick relevant parts from the examination of several systems in order to answer a question about the patient in front of you. Your task at medical school should be to learn to perform (fluently and thoughtfully) a full examination, systems examinations and cross-systems assessment of patients. This theme clusters some of these cross systems–assessments together.

These are actually quite complex; often there is no 'one right way' of conducting these assessments. To improve and develop in these patient assessments, you will need to apply a high level of thought before, during and after each assessment.

Requirements

Any willing patient will do, of course, although, as you become more confident, you may spend more time searching for the 'right' patients, whose signs will stretch your reasoning skills.

To improve, it is important that you get feedback from a member of staff or a colleague watching you. It is paramount to know where you doing well and where there is room for improvement. The complexity of these skills, and more than one right way to approach them, will make the feedback that you receive essential. Remember that different people will have different 'right ways'; your task is to consult widely and gain a consensus, without upsetting individuals.

30. Fluid status

Aims are to understand clinical assessment of fluid balance. To reinforce anatomy, physiology and good clinical practice. To begin to understand fluid balance in a clinical context. Some knowledge and clinical experience will be required so this will probably be suited to third year and above.

Perhaps a proforma/checklist can be produced.

Setting: Surgical ward (though learning opportunities can still be found on medical wards)

Activity: Choose five patients on which to assess fluid status. If possible be able to briefly examine the patient.

Charts:

Obs chart: HR, BP, temp, sats, RR. Look at current obs and review trends

Fluid chart: Calculate balance over last 3/7
~ fluid in: orally, IV fluid, meds and infusion, feeds
~ fluid out: urine, drains, NG tube, insensible loses (RR and temperature), stoma, aspirate, vomit, etc.

Fluid prescription chart: What has been prescribed and why?

Blood results: FBC, U+Es

Drug chart: Any drugs that could affect fluid balance and electrolytes. Any drugs that are potentially 'renal toxic' (NSAIDs, Abx, etc.)

Clinical

~ Skin turgor
~ Capillary refill/warmth of peripheries
~ Mucous membranes
~ Pulse (HR, volume and character)
~ Assess JVP
~ Check for peripheral oedema
~ Percuss and auscultate the lungs
~ Check catheter, stoma, drains (contents, are they open or closed?), NG tubes, infusions

Questions for students to answer

What are the average fluid requirements for an adult patient? What is the minimum urine output expected for an adult? Why is important to know the FBC and U+Es when assessing fluid balance and prescribing fluids/electrolyte replacement?

Is this patient clinically dehydrated, euvolaemic, fluid overloaded? What clues do you have to support your assessment of fluid status?

What fluids have been prescribed and why?

What would you suggest as the plan with respect to fluid balance for the next 24 hours for this patient?

Assessing fluid balance and prescribing fluid safely and effectively is one of the commonest things an FY1 will be expected to do.

Sameer Gujral, Doctor, UK

31. Speech and language therapy assessment

Physiotherapists and speech and language therapists can be really useful for teaching and observing SALT assessments on stroke wards and maxillofacial surgery/ head and neck surgery wards.

Ravinder Pabla, Doctor

An assessment of a patient's speech, language and swallowing requires you to think about the central nervous system (speech and language centres in the brain, cerebellar function, etc.), cranial nerves and structural problems in the mouth, pharynx, larynx, airways and oesophagus.

Reading about and then performing thoughtful speech and language therapy (SALT) assessments on a wide range of patients will help you revise your anatomy, physiology and pathology, as well as learning an important skill.

32. Is this patient well or ill?

Assessing whether a patient is well or ill (or becoming acutely unwell: 'going off') is one of the most important skills that you will learn. It will help you prioritise your workload as a junior doctor, and highlight to you when to call for help. There are various systems published (see further reading), the key point being that they involve a cross-systems assessment, not an end-of-the-bed glance!

The bored medical student should investigate the system in place within their specific Trust, for when a patient's systemic observations indicate that they should be reviewed by a senior doctor. There are various scoring systems used and each hospital will have it's own system in place.

The scoring system will indicate scores when the following observations are not within the 'normal limits' set out by the Trust: urine output (ml/h); systolic blood pressure (mmHg); heart rate (bpm); respiratory rate (rpm); oxygen saturation (%); temperature (°C); central nervous system response (e.g. gcs, avpu). For example, if a patient's respiratory rate is 26 rpm, then they will score on this observation, as their respiratory rate is not within 'normal' range.

If a patient scores above a certain number then this indicates they are 'at risk' and usually the procedure is for the staff nurse to alert the doctor. The 'early warning' or 'patient at risk' scoring system allows patients to be reviewed by a senior doctor earlier rather than later, and hopefully solves any problems before the patient becomes too unwell.

Some Trusts have an 'outreach team' which is made up of mainly ITU-based staff and they are on-call for when a patient becomes acutely unwell on the ward. The 'at-risk' scoring system will indicate with a high score when the patient should be seen by the 'outreach team' (if the Trust has one!) and they can intervene and give expert treatment to acutely unwell patients on the ward.

Rebekah Carter, Staff Nurse, UK

Theme: spot diagnosis

Background

One of the most rewarding things that you can do on the wards is to make instant spot diagnoses. Sometimes you will be right, sometimes you will be wrong, but that initial impression is an important one, and highly motivating when you get it right.

This involves some factual knowledge of clinical medicine and pathology, an eagle eye and a passion for curiosity.

When you think that you are right, check in the notes that you **are** right and then share your findings with others, if the patient is willing; other students may benefit. Clearly if you think that you have made a new diagnosis, missed by the clinicians caring for the patient, you should search them out and discuss the possibility with them.

When you are wrong, open the books and work out why, and head back to the patient. You will learn more by looking at why someone's signs **do not** fit into a pattern than you will from just learning stereotypes.

Requirements

It is worthwhile specifically mentioning consent here again. There may be times that you do not gain consent for spot diagnosis, e.g. looking out for abnormal gaits when walking down the high street, but these situations should be very rare indeed. If you are wandering on to a ward and trying to spot possible diagnoses from the ward entrance, make sure that you let the patients and the nurses know what you are doing first and check that it is OK with them. Clearly having two students stare at you from across the room and whisper to each other is likely to be seen as reflecting unprofessional behaviour.

Learning to recognise signs comes from examining patients – if you have seen five or ten patients with clubbing, you'll never miss the diagnosis in the future. Clearly, however, if you don't have a clue what clubbing, or Heberden's nodes or xanthelasma looks like you will stand little chance of spotting it! You may, therefore, want to spend some time on the tasks below.

Pick a condition from the ward round or just generally something you pick up on the wards. Go onto **www.google.com** and click on the search IMAGES sections. Type the name of the condition and search for images that come up. Pick some appropriate ones and paste them on a Microsoft PowerPoint slide. For example, if you type Addison's disease on Google, several pictures come up including pictures of pigmented skin, gums and a picture of John F Kennedy (because he suffered from Addison's). Paste these pictures together on one slide titled Addison's disease and move on to another condition. Gradually you will have several pictures for each condition and once you encounter another patient with a condition you have pictures for it – it makes it easier to recall and relate signs to patients.

Kumar Ahuja, Medical Student, UK

Construct a page detailing the common signs of illness which can be clearly seen just by looking at the patient's face, for example xanthelasma, blue lips (cyanosis etc.). Do the same for signs that can be seen in the hands...

Eimear O'Connor, Medical Student, Scotland

Theme: exploring around the patient

Background

History taking and examination of patients are, of course, core elements to clinical practice and crucially important skills to master during your medical training; the learning, however, doesn't have to stop there. So much more can be gained from your consultation with the patient. You also have the opportunity to explore a little about the patient and his or her story before and after the consultation.

Before even talking to the patient, a lot can be gained from pure observation. So often as a student, it is easy to rush into situations before taking time to think, but by practising skills of observation this allows you assess a situation, and gain knowledge of initial presentations of diseases. Similarly, after having gained a history from the patient (see Section 2 for how to take a history,) your knowledge can be built upon if you read around their illnesses.

Requirements

A patient's history, a pocket-sized medical textbook or access to the internet, a spare 10 minutes.

Use the patient as a 'hook'

The patient's story can become a basis on which you focus your learning. After you have a history from the patient, read around the disease with which he or she presented. Was the presentation typical? Did he or she have all the usual signs of that disease? By researching the pathology after you have seen a patient, it provides a face and presentation from which it is easier to recall the information. Having a face to put to the history and clinical signs elicited from that patient can act as a 'hook' on which you can place your knowledge of that disease.

Keep a copy of your favourite medical pocket book and start reading about cases available in the wards. If you have more time, take the history from the patient first and then read about the disease. Right now I'm on my first rotation for medicine and I'm using the Oxford Handbook of Clinical Medicine.

Afrah Mohammed, Medical Student, Saudi Arabia

Taking it a step further

Once you have read about the disease, and got to grips with the presentation of a certain condition, go on to look at investigations, management and treatments.

34. Observing from a distance

Take a chest X-ray from the patient notes trolley and look at it with your colleagues. Go through the motions of how to read the X-ray. Then come up with some possible differentials. This can be fun and each of you may have different ideas to throw into the ring. You can get clues to the diagnosis from looking for signs the patient has, i.e. nebuliser, oxygen mask, barrel chest, ECG monitor, type of cough, sputum pot and cigarette packets are all valuable clues. Remember that if observing from the end of the bed, explain what you are doing as the patient may seem mortified and perplexed as to why all eyes are on him/her! Finally look at the notes/X-ray report to see if you are correct. Even reporting on a normal chest X-ray is good practice.

Laura Geddes, Medical Student, UK

Spy on a patient and, simply by observing, see what signs they have – this is a good way to demonstrate that observation is the first thing you should do during any examination and you can miss a lot if you forget to look.

Amanda Jewson, Medical Student, UK

35. Guess the blood results

When on your paediatrics placement, go to the neonatal ward and have a look at each child in his or her cot. Try to guess the serum bilirubin level of the child based on the severity of jaundice. Then compare with the actual level on the blood results (usually found beside the cot). This is an excellent way of observing the levels of jaundice in neonates and recognising how the different skin tones of the neonates affects how much the jaundice is seen by the naked eye.

Tim Powell, Medical Student, UK

Revise how to check for conjunctival pallor correctly [see further reading], then go to the postnatal ward and guess a patient's haemoglobin level and then check in the notes – do it in twos or threes and engage the patients in the game (don't forget to introduce yourself to the midwives first). You will find a wide range of levels of anaemia, when you are way out, go back and have another look.

The student who guesses closest for each patient 'wins' a point; and the one with most points gets a prize! Don't forget to wash your hands.

Dason Evans, Doctor and Author

During my paediatrics rotation I found one of the most important and difficult skills to master was to answer the following questions
~ How old is the child?
~ How much do they weigh?
~ How tall are they?

There were all sorted of shocking and funny answers to these questions that we came up with.

Solution was just to go the end of the bed of many patients as there is time for (5 minutes per patient). Answering the questions above. Ask parents if you are right or look in the notes.

As a rough guide:
Weight (kg) = (age + 4) × 2
Height = 75 cm + (7 cm for each year above 1)

Hinesh Patel, Medical Student, UK

Taking it a step further

1. These examples are just a start of your training and development; you could make up plenty of other tasks around a spot diagnosis yourself.

2. Interestingly, there are several more accurate ways of assessing the level of anaemia than the usual glance in the eyes; why not try the task above after having done a PUBMED search on the topic. There have been some excellent meta-analyses. Keep a record of your successes and failures and see if you can beat published sensitivities and specificities for diagnosis of anaemia on clinical grounds!

References/further reading

Evans DE, Brown J (2009). *How to Succeed at Medical School: An essential guide to learning.* Oxford: Blackwell/BMJ Books.

Michels MEJ, Evans DE, Blok GA (2012). What is a clinical skill? Searching for order in chaos through a modified Delphi process. Medical Teacher, in press.

Sheth TN, Choudhry NK, Bowes M, Detsky AS (1997). The relation of conjunctival pallor to the presence of anemia. *J Gen Intern Med* **12**:102–6.

Early Warning Scores

You will find various published systems, here we list just a couple – a PUBMED search will reveal more.

Cooper N, Forrest K, Cramp P (2006). *Essential Guide to Acute Care.* Oxford: Blackwell/BMJ Books: Chapter 1.

Subbe CP, Kruger M, Rutherford P, Gemmel L (2001). Validation of a modified Early Warning Score in medical admissions. *Q J Med* **94**:521–6.

Section 4
PRACTICAL PROCEDURES

A person who never made a mistake never tried anything new.

Albert Einstein

Introduction

Clinical skills tend to include physical examination skills, communication skills and practical skills. We discuss physical examination skills in Section 3 and communication skills in Sections 2 and 6. Practical skills are sometimes divided into diagnostic skills (such as phlebotomy, lumbar puncture, ophthalmoscopy) and therapeutic skills (perhaps suturing, inserting a chest drain, catheterisation), although in reality many procedures sit within either classification depending on their context (e.g. aspirating a pleural effusion may be both diagnostic and therapeutic).

A more useful categorisation of practical procedures might be as follows:

1. Common tasks: the ones that, as a junior doctor, you will be likely to perform commonly (phlebotomy, cannulation, ophthalmoscopy, suturing).

2. Emergency tasks: the ones that you will need to be able to perform competently in an emergency situation (basic life support, defibrillation, performing a 12-lead ECG). These are particularly challenging because, by their nature, you will not have as much ongoing practice at them, but you will need to be highly proficient at the task when you do need to perform it.

3. Supervised tasks: the ones that you should be able to perform under supervision initially as a junior doctor (pleural tap, lumbar puncture).

4. 'Know about' tasks: the ones that you should know enough about to be able to explain what would be involved to a patient (barium enema, endoscopy).

5. 'Heard of' tasks: those rarer procedures that you should be able to recognise from a patient's description and know how do find out more information about (might include radiofrequency ablation of an osteoid osteoma).

Knowing what you need to be able to do, to what level

In the introduction to this book, we mention the importance of a portfolio. This should include a list of which different skills you need to know, to what level (1–5 above). This list can be built from various sources including your school's curriculum, the contents page of clinical skills books and national guidance (such as the GMC's

101 Things to Do with Spare Moments on the Ward, First Edition. Dason E Evans, Nakul Gamanlal Patel.
© 2012 Dason E Evans and Nakul Gamanlal Patel. Published 2012 by Blackwell Publishing Ltd.

'Tomorrow's Doctors' Document and the Scottish Doctor project). The list should include Practical Procedures, Physical Examination Skills, Communication Skills and even, perhaps, some deeper skills such as Clinical Reasoning. It is worthwhile reviewing this list often; remember that you will need to revisit skills often to become competent and then maintain competence.

How to learn a skill

In Section 3 we briefly discussed how to learn clinical/practical skills. Don't forget that learning a skill requires knowledge about that skill, practice and feedback (the Evans–Brown model, 2009). The knowledge required includes more than the steps that you will need to perform; it also includes the basic science behind those steps and the clinical reasoning that leads on from your findings (Michels et al. 2012).

Theme: know your equipment

Background

The first step in being able to perform a practical procedure is **not** knowing how it is done ('see one'), but relies on first knowing what equipment is required for each task, where it is kept, and how to check it and put any components together if required. Imagine that you have learnt how to carry out intravenous cannulation in the skills lab, but you do not know where the cannulas are kept on the ward, how to check that they are in date or how to tell a small-bore from a wide-bore cannula. Even if technically you can gain intravenous access, without this fundamental knowledge you would be pretty useless.

Similarly, even if you can take blood, would you know which bottle to use for a set of liver function tests? Clotting assessment? Antibiotic assay? α-Fetoprotein (AFP) estimation? Do you know how much blood should go into which bottle? There is often a preferred order for filling the bottles if multiple samples are required. Do you know what it is? How do paediatric bottles differ? What do blood culture bottles look like?

Requirements

Learning about equipment can be a convenient **thing** to do. There will be some occasions when you are feeling less sociable than usual, or some spare moments when you would prefer not to be seen. These are great times to make a trip to the equipment cupboard or a quiet corner of the ward.

As always, let one of the senior nurses know what you are doing, and if you would like to take any equipment away, make sure that you get permission to do so. The nurses may even know if there is any out-of date stock that is about to be destroyed; this would make great practice material. Also, you must know where and how you can safely discard any equipment once you have finished.

... one of the most important things I found out about hospitals was not knowing what each little bit of equipment was called or looked like. In [clinical skills] teaching we were introduced to a basic blood taking so I was familiar with the equipment I needed to take blood using a Vacutainer system. However, on many occasions syringes and needles, butterflies, cannulas, etc. are used, so it is a good idea if you are bored just to go to the equipment cupboard or room on the ward and just pick up (with clean hands of course) all the little bits of equipment and familiarise yourself with what they look like and what they are called. Such that if an SHO asks you to get a 'pink Venflon', for example, you are quick to get it and you know you have the right thing...

The same principle can be applied to different other pieces of equipment, i.e. catheterisation. On one occasion I was asked to get a size 12 Foley catheter. But when I went to the cupboard I did not know where to start looking or even what the equipment looked like.

So again, it would have been a great idea to just stay in a cupboard alone or with a friend and just go through the equipment and what it looks like and where to check for the sizes etc.

An even better idea would be to go home later and read about where you would use the various pieces in different situations; however, just knowing the various equipment pieces will save you a great deal of time and embarrassing moments.

Semeer Nakedar, Medical Student, UK

Taking it further

1. Familiarisation with equipment can go further than the ward equipment, of course. Manufacturers of medical instruments tend to design their equipment slightly differently to their competitors. It is therefore in your interest to 'play with' as many different sorts of ophthalmoscope, otoscope and doppler probes as you can find. Keep your eyes peeled for different models of equipment on the wards, in outpatients and general practice and, of course in the pockets or hands of your peers and members of staff. Spending a spare 2 minutes puzzling over how to turn on a Keeler otoscope can fill some spare moments on the ward, but spending the same time trying to work out how to switch it on in front of a patient or examiner can be deeply frustrating!

2. Theatres can also be a useful place to find out about equipment – both general (such as catheters, intravenous lines, cannulas) as well as specific surgical equipment (such as artery forceps, dissecting scissors, sutures).

37. Creative thinking

This ... idea is great for the 15 minutes or so between operations and has combined education and social benefits. When the scrub nurse wheels the instrument trolley away after an operation, follow them and say something like 'Excuse me, I'm the medical student and I wanted to learn about what you do as scrub nurses. Could you possibly run me through the names of some of the instruments?'.

~ They'll love you for showing interest in their job in a humble way (probably in complete contrast to the surgeon).

~ You'll learn the names of the instruments so you can get involved in handling instruments to a surgeon in theatre (massively impressive!).

~ Because the instruments are dirty, the nurse might let you handle them with a pair of gloves on while they tell you the instrument name and function. This is a great opportunity to figure out the mechanics and the feel of each instrument.

Umar J Wali, Medical Student, UK

For those who have a leaning toward engineering, or who have practical friends and family, why not spend some time considering how equipment might be improved. Often it is the 'shop floor workers' who can best spot opportunities for innovation, and this is one of the main directions of the current efficiency drives in the NHS. Sometimes the simplest suggestions have the largest impacts.

During my sessions in the clinical skills lab trying to train students on how to do endotracheal intubation... I noticed and observed one of them sitting alone with the tube in his hands and deeply distracted from class. One month later the student stepped forward and showed me how he could add fibreoptics to the tube to facilitate intubation instead of using the laryngoscope. He said why insist on using difficult procedures. Equipment difficult to use could be a rich substrate for students to examine and think [about] how to make easy. SOMETIMES!

Professor Omayma Aly, Egypt

It may sound basic, but most medical students and many junior doctors don't know how to operate hospital beds and couches. This results in them looking reasonably daft when a patient asks 'Can you give me a hand sitting up, doc?', and particularly stupid in clinical exams. More seriously, if you can raise the bed to the right height for a given task, then you are less likely to run into trouble with your back and neck later on in life, and you will be able to perform many procedures more safely. Most seriously, you will see colleagues trying to adjust beds, particularly outpatient couches, in ways that puts them at significant risk of major trauma to their arms or sometimes their heads!

Spend some time with different beds and couches experimenting ways to adjust them, offer to help nurses sit patients up at meal times on surgical and/or elderly care wards.

Experiment with the beds ... find out how the different ones work ... there's often too many buttons and sides and all the beds in the different hospitals work differently

Ruth Bird, Medical Student, UK

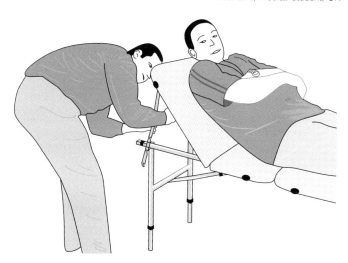

Taking it a step further

1. Back pain is one of the most common causes of time off work in the NHS, particularly of nurses. Simple training in manual handling techniques can have significant protective effects.

Look up the principles of manual handling – hopefully your school will have run some training, and both your library and the internet (occupational health and nursing sites in particular) will provide useful information. Convert the key principles into an observation checklist and use this to observe others on the ward. Identify common mistakes. You could even ask a peer to observe you in action using the same checklist.

39. Setting up an intravenous line

Intravenous (IV) infusions are often set up by the nurses on the wards, with junior doctors or senior medical students required to do so usually only in emergencies – the exact situations when it has to be right **first time, every time**. Although it looks easy, the process can be quite tricky, with risks including air embolus (unless you 'run through' properly), infection (so appropriate aseptic technique is essential) and spillage (the first time you try it – prepare to get wet, so use saline rather than dextrose, which can be sticky when it dries).

Ask a nurse to demonstrate either artificially (in side room) or by patient bedside, correct methods for setting up an IV giving set.

Intended learning outcomes:

~ Importance of checking patient identity, prescription and fluid (type, date)
~ Understand components of a giving set
~ Connecting fluid bag to giving set in a sterile way
~ How to run fluid through without making a mess! Importance of removing air bubbles
~ How to ensure fluid running
~ How to adjust rate of flow
~ Different types of fluids, their contents and situations in which they are prescribed

Use expired fluid/giving sets as does not use up essential resources.

Sameer Gujral, Clinical Teaching Fellow, UK

Taking it further

1. Think about the flow rate of different cannulas and giving sets. Imagine that you would like to give a litre of fluid to a patient as quickly as possible. How long would it take with each different combination? What would be the difference between a 'grey' and a 'green' cannula, for example? How about a giving set for 'blood' compared with a giving set for 'fluids'. Would one be better than the other?

2. If you can get hold of some out-of-date stock, why not give it a go and see how fast you can squeeze a bag of fluid through different combinations of giving sets and cannulas. Experiment: in an emergency when you need to give intravenous fluids quickly should you use a central line or grey cannula? Which is quicker? Is there much difference between a grey and a brown cannula? (It is probably worth doing outside on a summer's day, and be careful about disposal of sharps and the rest of the equipment because refuse collectors will assume that it is clinical waste and you might trigger an incident – so dispose of it appropriately!).

3. You will notice that different fluid bags contain different constituents; this might stimulate you to do some revision on fluid balance and indications, contraindications, cautions and prescription of fluids (see also Section 2)

> If there's a little bit of time to spare then taking IV fluid bags and doing some self-directed learning on fluids and electrolytes is a good learning opportunity. This is a topic students often get quizzed on and it is therefore good to review it, if only to remind ourselves about the different components.
>
> Sarah Onida, Medical Student, UK

See also

In Section 7 (Task 30) and Section 5 we talk about auditing case notes. You might apply what we write about audit to consider carrying out an audit related to equipment. Perhaps you could audit whether the clinical environment is stocked adequately to allow for safe venepuncture practice (see Schoeman et al. [2008] as a good example) or perhaps what proportion of staff have had manual handling training. If you do it well, and you have the right supervisor, then your results are likely to be useful and may even be publishable as a letter or presentable at a medical meeting – all of which are extra points for your CV.

Theme: peer practice of practical skills

Background

Peer practice has been central to medical training for hundreds, if not thousands, of years. In learning clinical skills, practising on each other usually follows practising in simulation and should usually precede practice with patients. Practising on your colleagues has benefits in improving fluency before practising with patients; it allows normal variations to be discovered and a clear understanding of the patient's perspective (unless you have had fundoscopy performed on you, for example, it will be difficult to know how uncomfortable it is or isn't as a procedure).

Requirements

You will need a peer and some equipment. It might be useful to have a second colleague to provide feedback, because 'patient' and 'clinician' can be so engaged with the task in hand that it becomes difficult to look in on the interaction 'from outside' and see what is really going on.

Essential to any peer practice is to obtain appropriate consent and have clear attention to 'patient's' dignity and confidentially; 'even though' it is practice on a peer, a focus on safety is crucial and excellent infection control is mandatory. We would recommend that you generate some brief ground rules between you (see Task 40).

40. Ground rules for peer practice

Negotiating ground rules for peer practice might sound a little obsessive, but read ahead for a moment before you rule it out.

Imagine that your colleague on the wards, someone you do not know well, got drunk and had a tattoo of Britney Spears put on his calf. He feels mortified about this and got teased about it at sixth form. Now he is at university he avoids sports and is careful in halls of residence to always wear tracksuit bottoms when walking about. Not knowing any of this, you ask him if you can practice feeling the pulses in his legs or checking his ankle–brachial pressure index (ABPI) using a handheld Doppler.

Clearly he will say no.

Imagine, however, if he knew and believed that you would treat him as respectfully as a patient, make every effort to ensure his privacy and maintain his confidentiality. Imagine that he knew that you would act professionally and that, when you saw the tattoo, you would acknowledge it – 'that's an interesting tattoo' – and, when he replied 'Ah, that's the biggest mistake of my life', you would say something suitable – 'It's funny, people seem to either love or hate their tattoos – I've never met someone who was indifferent!' – and then just move on professionally to continue with the task in hand. If he knew all this, that you would be as professional as the most professional doctor, do you think he would still say no?

This may seem like a daft example, but it is based on a true one. Other real examples include students who are self-conscious about scars (sometimes from surgery, burns or accidents, sometimes self-inflicted), about their weight (as you know, just because you think someone looks 'normal' doesn't mean that they see themselves as this in the mirror) and sometimes there are other reasons – gynaecomastia, being exceptionally ticklish – the list goes on!

In a spare 5 minutes when waiting for teaching on the wards, start a discussion with other students. Ask 'What could be students' concerns about peer practice' — make a list (abstracting this from personal to generic 'what **could** be ...' will allow a wider discussion). Get them to prioritise the list in two ways — which do they think are most common, which do they think are most important.

Consider the list and work out what you will need to **do** and what you will need to **say** in order to cover both the common and the important aspects. We have started a table as an example — it is incomplete:

Do	Privacy and dignity	Appropriate location Minimise risk of interruption (if in a side room tell nurses what you are doing and put a sign on the door etc.) Use gowns, even sheets of paper couch roll to maintain dignity
	Infection	Paper couch rolls for the examination couch for hygiene Ensure alcohol gel or sink is available; wash hands before and after Alco-wipes available to clean surfaces and any equipment
	Insert own ideas here	
Say	Confidentiality	'As I'm sure you know, I see examining a friend in the same way as examining a patient, so I might talk to other friends about what I learnt, but I will never talk about you and what I found'
	Privacy and dignity	'I'd like to be practising as if you are a real patient. Please let me know at any time if I should be covering you up more or if I forget something like making sure that the curtains are completely closed — it is really important that I learn these things. If you feel uncomfortable at any time, please let me know, I'll just stop'
	Insert own ideas here	

Taking it a step further

1. Keep a few pages in a notebook on the exercise above, and repeat the task as often as possible. Record how many students have input into the task, and note down when no new ideas seem to appear (this is referred to as 'reaching saturation' in qualitative research). You will steadily build a larger consensus on possible problems and their solutions. You may wish to speak to junior doctors about their opinions, or even senior doctors. How about nurses and physiotherapists – is there a difference?

2. Does your medical school have a formal written policy on peer physical examination (PPE)? If so, do your findings from your friends and colleagues match up?

3. What does the literature say? You will find a fair amount written on PPE – Charlotte Rees and Andy Wearn, among others, have researched into student views, and there is even a validated questionnaire that covers some aspects. Can you find PPE in medical ethics books? Is what they write about students examining patients relevant to students examining students?

4. Build a collaboration with some other students and a suitable member of faculty. Write up your findings from points 3, 2, 1 above and present it at the school. You may produce some useful guidance for future years. Who knows, it may even be publishable as a letter or an article in a journal.

5. We have already mentioned some validated questionnaires on PPE – would it be useful to apply one to your medical school? How about in collaboration with other medical schools? Talk to members of staff in clinical skills; this would make an interesting SSC or SSM (student-selected component or module).

---

41. Fundoscopy and otoscopy

These skills are often neglected by medical students, due partly to a perceived lack of availability of equipment, and partly to the fact that it takes quite a bit of practice before you start to be any good, and avoidance is often easier than feeling incompetent.

The ophthalmoscope and otoscope are sometimes missing from the ward or, more often, hidden somewhere to prevent them from going missing. Senior nurses (charge nurse or sister) may well be able to unlock the secret cupboard where they have guarded the equipment for years from theft. Make sure that you treat it with appropriate reverence and that you return it in perfect condition when you are done with it. If you leave it lying about, or give it to someone to pass on to someone else to give it to sister, then the next student along is less likely to get a favourable response.

Keep an eye on your colleagues' and junior doctors' pockets. Ask to borrow their equipment and write down their name and bleep. Make sure that you give it back to them in person, even if they have disappeared from sight and you are running late.

Ophthalmoscopy scares me and many of my friends. Use spare moments to really get to grips with how to handle one, including getting really close to your subject, and practise identifying the red reflex, scanning the four quadrants of each eye and hunting for the optic disc and macula.

Find yourself a darkened room (or lock yourself in the ward store cupboard, hoping no one puts two and two together and comes up with five!), and practise away.

When you feel confident with handling the scope and with identifying the optic disc and macula, try out your new skills on a patient or two. Work it into your standard neurological examination.

The more normal eyes you see, the more obvious an abnormality will be when you come across one.

Joanne Evans, Medical Student, UK

Outpatient clinics, A&E and general practice often have a set (ophthalmoscope and otoscope) bolted to the wall or on a large wheelie device – so if you can't find one on the wards, a trip to outpatients may be all you need to practise on a peer.

Taking it a step further

In general practice students have to wait for the GP to see the patient once they have finished their clerking. Students could use the time to practise their auroscope, ophthalmoscope and clinical examination skills.

Martin Mueller, GP Tutor, UK

1. The quote suggesting that ophthalmoscopy be added to a standard examination above makes two additional important points. With about 10 000 hours deliberate reflective practice required to become an expert in a skill, you will need to continue to practise for years. What better way than adding in a difficult skill to your routine examination procedure? In addition, we know that, if you don't use them, skills decay, so even if you are 'good enough' at a skill, you need to continue to use it, or you will loose it.

2. Are there truly no ophthalmoscopes on the wards? If so, why not work with some peers on an audit of ophthalmoscope availability. If fundoscopy is seen as an essential skill, and if practising fundoscopy is seen as essential for developing competence, then equipment should be available to allow practice. The medical school might be interested in the results of this audit.

For most babies that I examine I include fundoscopy. It is a difficult skill to perform in a baby, and once or twice a year these days it is essential that I can do it competently. I know that doing it once or twice a year is not enough to keep my skills up, so I add it to my routine examination.

Colin Stern, Consultant
Paediatrician, UK

3. Did you know that you can make your own lens-free ophthalmoscope for a few pounds/euros/dollars? Instructions on how to do so are in the public domain (Armour, 2000). They are not the same as the expensive models, but will get you used to navigating the retina and recognising normal and abnormal features.

See also
Task 6.

---

42. Phlebotomy and cannulation

An important note to be made here is that this should not be the first time for both students to be taking blood from someone. Someone there should be competent in the skills so as to know what to do at least. If in doubt just ask a house officer or even a nurse to watch you. It only takes a few minutes.

Sameer Nakedar,
Medical Student, UK

Phlebotomy and cannulation are key skills for junior doctors. With these skills being taken on more frequently by allied health professionals, often the junior doctor is asked to perform these skills either in an emergency or when the patient's veins are seen as difficult. In both these situations, you will need to be very good at the skill to succeed and, in both these situations, it is important that you succeed.

As always with peer practice, ensure that you have thought about safety aspects (Can you dispose of your sharps? What happens if the 'patient' feels faint?) and appropriate supervision.

I was appalled that some doctors had only performed one blood taking in medical school — one with an appalling excuse. If you haven't done one, see one, do one, teach one to a colleague. I am not ashamed to say I had two doctors watch my every move when taking blood for the first time but it really helped. Later in the year, I allowed my colleague to cannulate me, which greatly helped her confidence. Although I wouldn't recommend it to everyone, having someone watch you can be a great help and, when you get it right, sets you up for doing it yourself. Ask who needs bloods taken and don't be worried if you get it wrong or can't get any — try again on the next patient! You will become slick with the various methods of taking blood and it will prepare you for the OSCE exam.

Laura Geddes, Medical Student, UK

When bored on the wards and there are no jobs to do for the FY1s, ask a friend to practise putting Venflons in each other's arms. Make sure you get all the correct equipment; the person acting as the patient can help guide the student inserting the Venflon. This should only be done with medical students who aren't afraid of needles or who don't have a history of fainting easily. One you have had a go you can switch roles.

Daniel Braunold, Medical Student, UK

Taking it a step further
For those of you with a conscience.

Find a free anaesthetist, ideally one you have chatted with previously in surgery, and get them to administer a local anaesthetic on a fellow medical student. Then you can practise your first cannnulas/blood taking guilt free as you are neither practising on unsuspecting patients nor causing any pain to your mates. It may cost a couple of coffees later in the week as the bruise develops.

Claire Seeley, Medical Student, UK

See also
Other people's jobs, Task 87, Know your equipment, Task 36, Blood, Blood, Glorious Blood, Tasks 44 and 45.

ECG

ECG is another skill that is often performed by allied health professionals, but that as a junior doctor you will be expected to do quickly and competently in an emergency situation. You will therefore need to seize every opportunity going to practise this skill and make sure that you are 'slick' before you graduate.

43. Learning to record an electrocardiogram (ECG)

A common procedure students/doctors should know! Recording an accurate ECG integrates anatomical and physiological knowledge with clinical practice. It also allows students to reinforce clinical examination and communication skills.

With 'nothing' to do on the wards, this is a quick and useful exercise.

Most wards will have patients who require an ECG. Depending on the ward/equipment available this will be done be nursing staff or cardiology technicians who perform a daily ward round.

Students should ask nursing staff/cardiology technicians to learn how to perform a routine ECG. They can either assist or be directed to set up the equipment on a patient or another student (in a side/treatment room).

With appropriate explanation and consent, patients usually don't mind as this is a non-invasive harmless procedure.

Intended learning outcomes:

Basic

~ Placement of electrodes — practically and anatomically
~ How to ensure adequate contact from electrodes
~ Setting up an ECG machine
~ Instructions to patient to ensure best recording
~ What is an acceptable recording?
~ Ensuring ECG has patient name, DOB, hospital number, date, time recorded, including relevant clinical details (e.g. chest pain/ no chest pain)

Higher

~ Understanding of output — technical, i.e. rate 25 mm/s; layout of leads
~ Interpretation of ECG — normal and abnormal
~ When further action is required — indications to repeat ECG/ indications for thrombolysis
~ Other relevant cardiovascular investigations

(Encourage students to seek out local protocols — forms on ward/intranet)

Sameer Gujral, Clinical Teaching Fellow

Taking it a step further

1. An ECG is an excellent opportunity to revise your surface markings of the chest. Work with an anatomy book and a peer, possibly with a pen (if they don't mind being drawn on) in order to be certain that you can identify the key anatomical points and planes and what underlying structures they relate to. Consider how you might place the electrodes if a patient had situs inversus/dextrocardia. How about pectus excavatum? How would you document any adaptation from standard ECG placement in the notes?

2. Review the theory behind ECG – remind yourself of the electrophysiology. What does each part of the trace tell you? Use these basic principles to consider how misplacement of the leads or stickers might lead to an apparently abnormal trace. Now try this on a colleague – see if you can generate an 'abnormal' ECG by making technical errors. Think about what implications this has for your future practice in both taking and interpreting an ECG.

3. How many leads does the standard '12-lead' ECG require? Why? For those thinking about a career in cardiology/intensive care, have a look for articles on 15- and 18-lead ECG traces.

See also

Data interpretation (ECG) – Section 7, Tasks 80 and 81, Hidden teachers (ECG) – Task 46.

Theme: hidden teachers, hidden opportunities for practical skills practice

Background

Even though you may be attached to a certain team of doctors on the wards, there are plenty of other people around with the expertise and time to teach or supervise you. Finding these hidden teachers can be one of the most significant things that you can do to improve your learning on the wards (probably coming third after learning to work with other medical students and seeing lots of patients). We have clustered quite a few submissions here, but you may wish to start your own list. Speak to students who have been on your placement before, and those who are or have been at your hospital or clinic – senior students will be particularly useful – and see if you can build an inventory of places to go and contacts.

Requirements

The most essential requirement is an appropriate approach. In general most people want to teach. People tend to enjoy teaching keen students; it makes most people feel warm, like you have done some good today. Dealing with rude, demanding or disinterested students has the opposite effect. For some readers this will be so obvious that you will be frustrated that we are writing it. For others, this will be big news. These students believe that it is their right to be taught, and that they should demand teaching at every opportunity. These students tend to get rapidly disenchanted with the clinical learning environment, and become rather bitter that other students get more teaching, but, when they demand it, everyone seems too busy.

Consider your approach to asking others to teach you. If you ask with a smile, if you make clear that you are asking because you are keen to learn, and if you take a 'no' graciously, your chance of getting a 'yes' will be much higher and your morale won't be so affected if you get a 'no'. Practise asking by role-playing with your peers, and practise how you will respond to various answers. For example, to 'No, I'm far too busy' you might respond 'OK, of course, no problem. Is there anything I can do to help like [take forms to radiology/write blood forms/add relevant]?'

Think about how you might try to be useful to the people who are teaching you. Imagine, for example, that you spend half a day with the ECG technicians in cardiology outpatients (see Task 43), you prepared in advance, and you were keen and enthusiastic. You watched them take a few outpatient ECGs and then you did a couple under supervision, and by the end of the morning you were able to do it with minimal supervision. Chances are that the technicians were running late because of you, and may have missed out on their usual coffee break or some of their lunch because they were teaching/supervising you. They might not mind because you were a pleasure to have around, and they think that they may have done some good in helping you learn. Imagine now that you go back on another couple of half-days to help out. They will need to supervise you less, and so will be able to get through patients more quickly (many hands make light work, and all that); in addition you will get faster and gain experience with a wider variety of patients, there will always be someone there to ask for help if you run into a challenge, and they are likely to grab the 'keen medical student' if there is something interesting happening. Everybody wins.

On a similar note, the student who 'mucks in' – makes the tea, cleans up the rubbish, brings biscuits – is likely to be seen more positively than the one who looks like he or she is too important.

When you make good contacts, consider how you will keep them open. Think about sending them a thank-you email or thank-you card, or even dropping them an email once a month, letting them know how you are getting along. Chocolates are always welcome. You may wish to ask if it would be alright to come back and see them if you run into problems in the future, and perhaps asking permission to tell other students about what a fantastic learning opportunity this was.

If 'cheek and charm' doesn't come naturally to you, spend time consciously working on it. Identify others who **do** have the skills you want to learn and talk to them, watch them, keep notes. Consider not only their behaviour (what they say to people, what non-verbal communication they use) but also their attitude to learning and how these behaviours and attitudes compare with your own. You will gain a lot by asking a simple open question such as 'You always seem so enthusiastic, what do you do when you have off days?' and just being curious about their response.

44. Blood, blood, glorious blood

Phlebotomy and cannulation feature very highly in submissions for this book. This probably reflects the facts that these are common tasks for senior medical students and junior doctors, they are not always easy tasks to begin with (there is quite a steep learning curve), and, as they are invasive and, indeed, painful procedures, it is important to climb that steep learning curve as quickly and with as much good supervision as possible.

Phlebotomists are a fantastic resource. They are experts in their field and tend to always use best practice when taking blood, unlike some doctors. As such they make excellent teachers and fantastic role-models. You may wish to work with the phlebotomists when you are a novice, and again when you think that you are reasonably good. The phlebotomists will be able to show you how to take blood in a safe way from patients with difficult veins. Later on in life, you will be able to pass this information on, and may help prevent other students and doctors from suffering a needlestick injury.

In the third year, when nothing was happening on the ward, I would go down to the pathology department and ask a phlebotomist if they needed a hand so that I could practise venepuncture. The first time I went, they watched me for the first few times to make sure I was safe and knew what I was doing. Then they would let me help with their list. Brilliant way to practise.

Anushka Aubeelack, Medical Student, UK

Some hospitals specifically have medical student phlebotomy sessions in the phlebotomy clinic, which you can book into; others rely on students who are proactive to make contact. In some situations, particularly if you are in a busy teaching hospital, you may find that the phlebotomy clinic is not welcoming to students, but, if you don't ask, there will be no way of knowing! Phlebotomists also come onto the wards, usually for a morning 'blood round'. The timing of the rounds depends on the hospital and the ward involved.

For third-year medical students, or finalists who want practice: contact the phlebotomists in the morning, and tell them you'd like to practise taking bloods. Follow them on their ward rounds, and do their bloods for them! You get loads of practice, and even more satisfaction when your Vacutainers start filling! Much better than rubber arms.

Daijun Tan, Medical Student, UK

When there is nothing to do on the ward, a couple of times I went to the phlebotomy clinic and practised taking blood there to make use of my time. Found it very useful and indeed became more confident in my practical skills. And at times I went to the medical assessment unit to practise cannulation and ABGs.

Ali Al-lami, Medical Student, UK

Junior doctors, of course, will be grateful for assistance in everyday jobs, and you can use that to your advantage.

45. Taking a history while the blood bottle fills

Housemen [FY1s/interns] everywhere are overworked — asking them if they need any help with taking the bloods will definitely be met with a yes. Ask if you can be sent to an interesting case.

Utilise the time with the patient well — take a history while preparing the bottles, and then assess why each sample is being taken in relevance to the case. This way, history taking, thought process and phlebotomy skills are all being exercised at the same time. Plus, the houseman will be thankful for it! Just watch out for needlestick injuries.

Paul Cacciottolo, Medical Student, Malta

In addition to the wards, phlebotomists in the ward and phlebotomy clinic, and the medical assessment unit (MAU), other popular locations submitted by students include the haematology day unit, the day surgery unit and A&E. Do not forget that many general practices run phlebotomy clinics too.

As a medical student you cannot get enough practice at practical procedures under supervision so that when you are a junior doctor the ordeal of everyday tasks in your working life will not seem as daunting. A good tip is to make friends with an anaesthetist, get their theatre list for the next day and go with them to see preoperative patients. While you are doing this, ask for the patients' fully informed consent for you to perform some practical procedures in the anaesthetic room, such as inserting Venflons or catheters, if required. The anaesthetist and anaesthetic nurse do so many of these types of procedures in the day they will likely be only too glad to let you help out.

Alison Bradley, Medical Student, UK

Taking it a step further

1. You may have noticed in the introduction to this theme, and during Task 44 that we highlight the importance of safe practice in taking blood. Unsafe practice is common on the wards. Spend some time listing all the steps that you can go through to ensure safety. This might include safety for the patient (checking identity and labelling appropriately, ensuring that equipment is sterile and in date, ensuring appropriate consent), safety for you (how do you minimise or even negate risk of needlestick injury, splash injuries, etc.?) and safety for others (sharps disposal, not walking across the wards with sharps, ensuring there is no spillage, etc.).

Compare this list with what you will find in the literature, and ask some experts (perhaps phlebotomists, occupational health personnel, head of clinical skills at your medical school) to look through and critique it. What have you left off? This is an easy **thing** to do in spare moments, writing down your thoughts in the back of a notebook until you have a comprehensive list.

See also
Peer practice – Tasks 40 and 42, Knowing equipment – Task 36.

46. Learning practical skills from and with other professions

Overview

Doctors and phlebotomists are not the only people with things to teach. This collection of tasks introduces just some of the people who others have found useful in providing teaching and experience for students. It would be worth casting some thought to Section 6. Interprofessional education can sometimes have a bad reputation, but imagine that, in addition to learning some skills, you also learn about what it is that nurses, ECG technicians, phlebotomists, physiotherapists, occupational therapists etc. actually do (and don't do), and you learn how to work with them effectively. Once you graduate, life as a junior doctor will be so much easier for you!

So you went in early only to realise that your consultant's theatre list was cancelled, and there were already three students sitting in the clinic, you've done 10 clerkings since Monday and it's only Wednesday, and there's no ward round.

Head off to any of the theatres, grab an **anaesthetist** and tell him/her that you would love to learn something and stick around for, say, half a day (as Wednesday afternoons are for sports). Anaesthetists are one of the friendliest bunches in the medical world, and they are the best people to teach practical stuff like cannulation, airway management or even the theory side — physiology, fluid management, etc. Just anything. Most of them are happy to teach, and let you practise (on consenting patients) under their supervision. So there you go, one whole morning (i.e. half a day) you probably get to put in four Venflons and intubate three patients. If you're a third year and doing your attachment in a super busy hospital where everyone can't wait to get rid of you, that's awesome.

Ying Ci Ng, Medical Student, UK

From my previous experience in the NHS I often found it very useful spending time with other specialties when I had a free moment. This allowed me to better understand their roles, which in turn allowed me to refer patients more appropriately. There are various skills possessed and tasks performed by other health professionals which I think doctors are completely unaware of/ have no idea how to go about performing these tasks, if required. Something I came across frequently was a doctor's inability to safely observe a patient's mobility on the ward, i.e. they had poor manual handling and lacked skills to help facilitate the patient's mobility. Often I heard them saying to a patient 'Let's have a look at your mobility then' but didn't take the time to acknowledge that the patient may be at a very early in their stage of rehab from a mobility point of view.

Asheesh Bharti, Medical Student, UK

Go to the reception desk/nurse in charge and ask them for the bleep number for the **thrombolysis nurse**. Or alternatively find out where he/she can usually be found.

Talk with them and shadow them for a few hours. The chances are that they will teach you how to do ECGs (watch one, do one) and then they will also teach you how to interpret them.

The one time I did this in A&E, the thrombolysis nurse gave me a step-by-step guide of first doing the ECGs and then interpreting them. They've usually got a lot more time, patience and enthusiasm to teach as this is completely their area of expertise. In the few minutes, or hours, that you spend with them, you will learn so much.

The more time you spend with them, the more grounded your ECG skills will become.

Sharavanan Jeyanathan, Medical Student, UK

At 8am, 2pm or later as required, why not complete a set of observations on a patient at a time when they would need them taken by a healthcare assistant anyway. This will be good practice on observation taking, get to know a patient better, good to go and review the basic physiology. It will also be helpful for the care assistant or nurse if you let them know you are doing it; it may save them some work.

Sian Low, Medical Student, UK

If you find that your ward is quiet or if you have a few spare minutes or hours, why not call into the acute receiving ward? If you show up there with sleeves rolled up volunteering to do bloods, Venflons, arterial blood gases, blood cultures, ECGs, etc. (provided you are at a stage of training where you are competent in these tasks) they might just hug you there and then! Seriously, though, as

*a student learning to perform such tasks in a pressured environment
and getting practical experience this is a great experience.*

Alison Bradley, Medical Student, UK

Taking it a step further

These examples are the tip of the iceberg. Spend some time thinking about the other professions in the hospital, and what you might learn from them. Discuss this with your peers and junior doctors; see whom you have left off. You might carry around this list on a page in your notebook, so that when you come across another profession that you are curious about you can add them to the list. In this current clinical attachment, see how many of these different professionals you might shadow and, at the end of the attachment, spend some time noting down what you learned (perhaps in your portfolio), and who else you will need to find out about during your next attachment.

Related tasks

Tasks 70 and 66.

Theme: infection control

Background

Nosocomial infections are common, and can be devastating. MRSA (methicillin-resistant Staphylococcus aureus) and *Clostridium difficile* are high-profile infections, but it is worthwhile remembering that healthcare-acquired infections include a wide range of other problems such as wound infections, pneumonias, and gastroenteritis. Historically, as far back as 1847, hand washing in attending clinical staff was shown to reduce sepsis and mortality in postpartum women, and yet, even today, hand-washing practice leaves much to be desired. What better way to spend your spare moments on the ward than ensuring that you do not pass infections on from one patient to another?

We estimate that 1.7 million HAIs [hospital-acquired infections] occurred in U.S. hospitals in 2002 and were associated with approximately 99,000 deaths. The number of HAIs exceeded the number of cases of any currently notifiable disease, and deaths associated with HAIs in hospitals exceeded the number attributable to several of the top ten leading causes of death reported in U.S. vital statistics.

These estimates are sobering and reinforce the need for improved prevention and surveillance efforts.

Klevens et al. (2007)

47. Now wash your hands

Find a poster on hand washing on the ward, look at your notes or have a look on the internet (UK Department of Health, World Health Organization, UK NHS, nursing and a wide range of other reputable websites) and write down all the steps that you need to go through. Find a sink and someone to watch you, and wash your hands. Ask them to score you on your list of steps – how did you do? If you made mistakes, do it again, and again, until you get it right each and every time

When I was a new hospital chaplain, no one showed me how to wash my hands, but I realised it was important. I found a sink with a poster on hand washing over it, and practised and practised. When I thought I could do it well, I asked one of the nurses to watch me and tell me if I was up to scratch.

I wash my hands before I go and see each patient, and after I have finished with them. Sometimes I notice that other health professionals seem to forget.

Peter Cowell, Hospital Chaplain, UK

Taking it a step further

1. It is likely that you have had some training in hand washing. Skills labs often have invisible gel or powder that fluoresces under UV light. Why not book up a session in the skills lab and check to see whether your technique gets rid of all the gel (and hence would get rid of any infection)? Often there is an area that you might have missed. Do it several times and try and be as real to life as possible (your usual 'quick' hand wash).

2. Washing your hands right while the focus is on hand washing is one thing, doing it right in practice another. Talk to the other students on attachment with you, share your checklist for hand washing that you wrote above, and ask them to watch you when you are not expecting it. Do you follow the WHO five moments for hand hygiene (see the figure)? Do you wash all areas of your hands for the right length of time?

3. Of course, the same goes for alcohol hand-rub. Do you know when it should and shouldn't be used? How much should you use? How should you rub it around your hands? We have seen lots of people applying homeopathic doses of alcohol to the palms of their hands, rubbing palms briskly together – which makes us wonder why they bothered. We've seen others applying large quantities of alcohol gel to their hands and then wiping it off on the seat of their trousers.

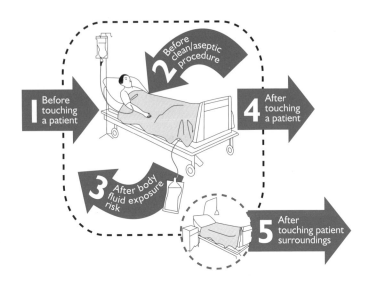

48. It's not just your hands

The stethoscope as a vector of infection (or not) ...

~ Take a look at the head of your stethoscope.
~ How clean does it look?
~ Does it matter?

Go and get a couple of alcohol swabs (injection site swabs) and clean the diaphragm and bell of your stethoscope while thinking about the second question. Now find a PC with internet access and perform a search to find an answer to the question.

Andy Wearn, Clinical Senior Lecturer, New Zealand

Taking it a step further

I. In a spare moment write an inventory of equipment carried by junior doctors, nurses and other members of the healthcare team. This might include stethoscopes, ophthalmoscopes, tourniquets, fob watches, pens, even ID swipe cards. For each of these items, imagine how they might transmit infection from one patient to another. For example, does one of the other medical students on your attachment turn the ophthalmoscope on, then hold the patient's head or eye open (not good practice), then switch the ophthalmoscope off, all with the same thumb? Does he or she wipe the instrument with an antiseptic wipe?

2. Spend some time with the nurses cleaning and decontaminating empty patient beds. Not only will you become more popular with the nurses, but you will learn what they do to clean around the bed area when one patient leaves, before another arrives. While you are cleaning the bed, consider the parts that are difficult to clean, generally get missed out or impossible to reach without a steam cleaner. Consider what implication this might have for nosocomial infections if there is a high turnover of patients.

3. Does your hospital Trust have a bare-below-the-elbow policy? How well is it adhered to? How is it enforced? What can a literature search tell you about the infection risk associated with wrist watches, shirt cuffs or ties? The infection control team and/or microbiologists may be looking for someone to help with an audit or even some research to fill the gaps in the literature.

4. For those particularly interested in cultural diversity, what policy does your hospital or medical school have for students and staff whose personal or religious beliefs are not consistent with 'bare below the elbow'? How is the policy or lack of policy that you find justified?

See also
Audit and Research within Section 7.

References/further reading

Armour RH (2000). Manufacture and use of home made ophthalmoscopes: a 150th anniversary tribute to Helmholtz. *BMJ* **321**:1557–9.

Evans DE, Brown J (2009). *How to Succeed at Medical School: An essential guide to learning*. Oxford: Blackwell/BMJ Books.

Health Protection Agency Centre for Infections (2009). *Healthcare-associated Infections in England: 2008–2009 Report*. London: Health Protection Agency.

Klevens MR, Edwards JR, Richards CL, et al. (2007). Estimating health care-associated infections and deaths in U.S. hospitals, 2002. *Public Health Rep* 122.

Michels MEJ, Evans DE, Blok GA (2012). What is a clinical skill? Searching for order in chaos through a modified Delphi process. Medical Teacher. in press.

National Audit Office (2003). *A Safer Place to Work: Improving the management of health and safety risks to staff in NHS Trusts*. London: National Audit Office.

Nicol M (2000). *Essential Nursing Skills*, Edinburgh: Mosby.

Schoeman S, O'Connor EF, Harrison R, Muirhead-Smith A, Shah MA, Ware N (2008). Venepuncture technique training vs practice: a survey of foundation year 1 doctors. *Br J Hosp Med (Lond)* **69**:524–8.

World Health Organization (2009). WHO Guidelines on Hand Hygiene in Health Care (First Global Patient Safety Challenge Clean Care is Safer Care). Geneva: WHO. See 'My 5 moments for hand hygiene'. Available at: www.who.int/gpsc/5may/background/5moments/en/index.html.

General Medical Council. (2009). *Tomorrow's doctors: Outcomes and standards for undergraduate medical education*: General Medical Council.

Simpson JG, Furnace J, Crosby J, Cumming AD, Evans PA, Friedman Ben David M, et al. (2002). The Scottish doctor–learning outcomes for the medical undergraduate in Scotland: a foundation for competent and reflective practitioners. *Med Teach* **24**(2):136–143.

In addition:

An anatomy book of your choice.

A practical ECG book that explains how and why to place electrodes (the nursing section of the library will be useful here).

A basic ECG interpretation book.

Section 5
PRESCRIBING

With contributions from Ammy Lam

… it usually requires a considerable time to determine with certainty the virtues of a new method of treatment and usually still longer to ascertain the harmful effects.
Alfred Blalock 1899–1964

Introduction

49. Pharmacology in practice

Pharmacology is very important in medical practice but can be one of the least taught subjects in medical school. A good understanding of the mechanism of action, indications, contraindications and cautions, and adverse effects of common drugs is an essential prerequisite to good medical prescribing. While most pharmacology knowledge can be taken directly from a textbook, by linking pharmacology to actual real-life patients, you are more likely to remember and understand the reasoning behind why drugs are prescribed.

Mosaab Aljalahma, Medical Student, Kuwait

Prescribing is one of the most common practices carried out by doctors. A sound knowledge base of important aspects of medications form an essential part of a doctor's armamentarium. In addition, monitoring of side effects and appropriate patient counselling need to be considered. A separate section on errors is included given the fact that the National Patient Safety Association (NPSA) has highlighted the need to reduce the number of preventable medication errors, which remains high.

50. 'BRAINS & AIMS'

Apply the following mnemonic, 'BRAINS & AIMS', to any medications that you 'aim' at your patient.

101 Things to Do with Spare Moments on the Ward, First Edition. Dason E Evans, Nakul Gamanlal Patel.
© 2012 Dason E Evans and Nakul Gamanlal Patel. Published 2012 by Blackwell Publishing Ltd.

BRAINS & AIMS gives key principles of WHAT you should learn about/know about each drug, for WHICH drugs if students want a list of 'Top 100 Drugs' prescribed by foundation doctors, see Baker et al. (2011) paper.

Benefits	Benefits to this patient
	Benefits to the wider population (e.g. herd immunity)
	Benefits to the health service (e.g. cost)
Risks	Risks to the patient
	Risks to others (e.g. cytotoxics)
Adverse effects	Generally common and mild
	Also consider the rare but serious
Interactions	Interactions with things patient is currently taking
	Also potential interactions that you should warn about
Necessary prophylaxis	Prophylaxis of potential adverse effects (e.g. additional drugs where necessary – PPI cover for NSAIDs)
Susceptible groups	Such as elderly people, pregnant women, patients with pre-existing renal/liver disease
Administration	What choices do you have?
	What if the patient can't take tablets or is a vegan?
Information	What key information should you explain to the patient?
Monitoring	Should you monitor for action of the drug?
	For adverse effects?
	Monitor drug levels?
Stopping	Is this drug for life?
	If not what is your plan for stopping?
	How will you make this plan clear to the patient and in the patient record?

Reproduced courtesy of Dr Andrew Webb, Senior Lecturer/Honorary Consultant in Cardiovascular Clinical Pharmacology, Kings College London/Guy's and St Thomas' NHS Foundation Trust, London.

This can be used before prescribing or terminating a patient's medication. It helps appropriate prescribing and prevents potential errors.

Theme: navigating around the drug chart

Background

Doctors of all grades use drug charts and prescribe regularly, and this is more frequent when you first start as a junior doctor. The drug chart is one of the most important patient documents that you will use.

Despite, or perhaps because of its frequency of use, it remains one of the most common sources of medical error (Tasks 54 and 55 give further information).

Drug charts are used as a means of communication between healthcare professionals, usually between doctors, pharmacists and nurses. Very often, medication errors and subsequently patient harm occurs when there is a breakdown in communication, in this case usually as a result of unclear or incorrect prescribing on the drug chart. It is therefore crucial that prescribers are familiar with what they are prescribing on and signing for. There are many variations in the way that drug charts are laid out and you will find that each hospital does it slightly differently. The same hospital may even have different charts for different patient populations, e.g. ITU drug chart vs general ward drug chart vs paediatric drug charts, or separate charts for diabetic medications, fluids, epidurals, anticoagulation. To find out what your hospital uses, speak to your ward pharmacist. They can go through nitty gritty rules of prescribing and explaining the layout of drug charts. This will help ensure that you prescribe safely to protect yourself and the patient.

Ammy Lam, Principal Pharmacist for Surgery and Critical Care,
Barts and The London Trust

Requirements

Familiarising yourself with drug charts is an excellent use of time. It will not only be useful during your time as a medical student but also help once you graduate and improve your understanding of prescribing.

Depending on the task that you attempt to carry out, you may need as little as a blank drug chart. If you are feeling much more sociable, you may need an amenable patient, his or her drug chart and medical notes, a BNF (*British National Formulary*), and an approachable doctor or pharmacist.

Once again, if you are going to be using any charts or notes that belong to a patient, you must notify the relevant clinical staff. You must also gain informed consent to talk to a patient before starting a consultation (see page xii of the introduction). If you decide to practise using drug charts then you must draw a line across it and clearly write 'practice' across all its pages in bold writing to prevent this being confused

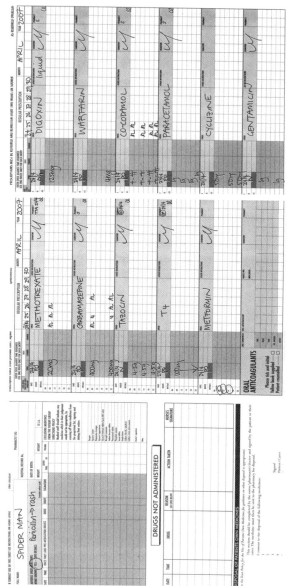

Standard drug chart (inside). Used with permission from Barts and The London NHS Trust.

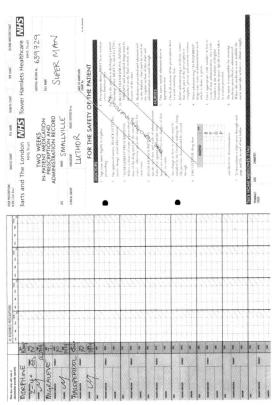

Standard drug chart (back page, cover). Used with permission from Barts and The London NHS Trust.

with a real patient's chart. Obviously ask permission from the ward staff before taking a blank chart away to practise with.

51. Know your way around drug charts

Although this sounds like a relatively simple task, you will find that all Trusts have different styles of presenting their drug charts. Most have the same headings (patient details, regular medication, allergies, once-only medication, as required medication, etc). Knowing the layout and sections of the chart will help you prescribe safely and swiftly.

Pick up a blank drug chart and read through all the headings to see if you understand what each one means. Can you think of examples of drugs that can be prescribed on each of these sections?

Taking it a step further

1. Ensure that you navigate your way around as many different drug charts as possible. Ask your friends studying at different hospitals to collect drug charts and then you can compare how these vary. For example, some drug charts may have enoxaparin and TEDS (thromboembolic deterrent stockings) already printed on the charts and have to be signed for or crossed out. Can you think why this might be?

2. Often there are several different drug charts: standard, intensive care, diabetic (see figure below), fluid, anticoagulation, paediatric. See if you can obtain these and discuss with a friend/doctor/pharmacist/nurse why they might vary. This may also give you an opportunity to travel around the hospital.

52. Patient-centred pharmacology self-teaching

There is no better way to learn pharmacology than to see it in a clinical context. You are much more likely to remember and retain this knowledge for the future.

Take a patient's drug chart and list the medications they are on. Make a list of the indications for each drug used and then deduce a differential diagnosis list for the patient based on their current medication.

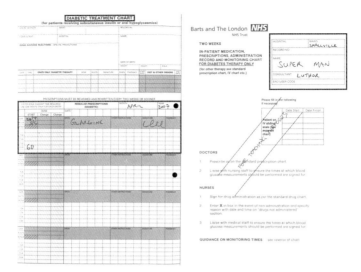

Diabetic drug chart (back page, cover). Used with permission from Barts and The London NHS Trust.

Justify your differential list by explaining why the patient's drug would be used to treat the conditions in the list (i.e. pharmacodynamics and mechanism of action)

Note any contraindications and/or cautions of the patient's drugs

Make a list of possible adverse effects due to the patient's drugs

Talk to the patient after introducing yourself and obtaining verbal consent. Focus on the patient's presenting complaint, past medical history and drug history. Use the chat to confirm or rule out your differential diagnosis list, and also explore if any of the side effects you thought of were experienced by the patient. Does the patient report anything that was in your contraindications list?

Use your patient interview and the BNF to review the notes you made before talking to the patient.

Identify any errors or weaknesses in your knowledge and revise using a pharmacology textbook.

Mosaab Aljalahma, Medical Student, Kuwait

Taking it a step further

If, in the future, the patient's medications or dosages are changed, make a list of possible reasons why this was done (ordered from most likely to least likely). Then confirm by talking to the patient or discussing this with the senior doctor, or both.

Mosaab Aljalahma, Medical Student, Kuwait

53. 'Re-boarding'

This can be one of the most common requests from nursing staff or pharmacists to junior doctors. **Re-boarding** simply refers to the process of rewriting the drug chart and adjusting as appropriate for medications that are no longer required, adjusting doses, addition of new medication, etc.

The task can become mundane for most juniors and any help in re-boarding

'Can you come and **re-board** this drug chart, doc?'

The first time I was asked to **re-board**, I didn't have a clue what I was being asked! I was scared.

Identity withheld, Junior Doctor, UK

can be of great assistance to the already stretched doctor. Of course, you must not sign for the drugs; this is still the legal responsibility of the doctor. This can be a fantastic opportunity to learn and be helpful – two for the price of one!

Rewriting a full drug chart at the end of the week endears you to both nurses and house officers especially if you have neat handwriting.

Ruth Heseltine, Medical Student, UK

Taking it a step further

Look through the medications on it [drug chart you have just re-boarded]. Then, sit somewhere with the BNF and read about the drugs, and think about why they may have been used. When done, and if confident in your reading ability, try to formulate why that drug is being used, i.e. the condition the drug is being used to treat. When done, flick through the patient's notes and see if

you were correct (check the PMH or current problem list).
Repeat for x number of patients.

Junaid Campwala, Medical Student, UK

Work out what they all are [patients' medications], how they work, two side effects and why the patient is on each of the drugs. Very easy and surprisingly useful. Anything you're not sure about you can ask one of the doctors.

Emily Chung, Medical Student, UK

Theme: preventable human errors in prescribing

Background

Medication error refers to 'any preventable event that may cause or lead to inappropriate medication use or patient harm while the medication is in the control of health professional, patient or consumer …' (originally from National Coordinating Council for Medication Error Reporting and Prevention, see Further reading).

Every day, an average hospital administers about 7000 medicine doses. Nurses spend 40% of their time administering medicines. NHS staff reported almost 60 000 medication incidents to the NPSA over an 18-month period. It is estimated that 7% of inpatients may suffer harm from medicines, much of which is preventable. That means that, for every 14 patients whom you see, one of them will suffer harm from medication errors. That's more that one per average-sized ward! Can you spot the medication errors on your ward?

Requirements

Again you will require patient's drug chart and medical notes, a BNF, and an approachable doctor or pharmacist.

---

54. Spotting medication errors

In order for you to appreciate the kinds of mistakes that can occur on drug charts, below is an example of a drug chart with several errors. This is our example; why not write your own (make sure that you cross through the pages so that it is clear that its for teaching purposes only).

See how many medication errors you and your peers can find. Have a prize for the one that can spot the most

Ammy Lam, Principal Pharmacist for Surgery and Critical Care, UK

Find the medication errors.

FULL NAME: SPIDER MAN

Penicillin→rash

DRUGS NOT ADMINISTERED

DISPOSAL OF PATIENT'S OWN MEDICINES

ORAL ANTICOAGULANTS

REGULAR PRESCRIPTION MONTH APRIL YEAR 2007

DIGOXIN liquid

WARFARIN

CO-CODAMOL

PARACETAMOL

CYCLIZINE

GENTAMICIN

METHOTREXATE

CARBAMAZEPINE

TABOON

T4

METFORMIN

Here are the answers.

FULL NAME: SPIDER-MAN   Wrong patient

Penicillin → rash   Non-capital letters

DRUGS NOT ADMINISTERED

DATE	TIME	DRUG	REASON NOT GIVEN	ACTION TAKEN	NURSE'S SIGNATURE

Non completed

DISPOSAL OF PATIENTS OWN MEDICINES

ORAL ANTICOAGULANTS

REGULAR PRESCRIPTION — MONTH: APRIL   YEAR 2007

METHOTREXATE   Wrong frequency

Wrong timing   Incorrect timing

CARBAMAZEPINE   Missed dose

TAZOCIN   Allergy

T4   Incorrect timing

METFORMIN   Abbreviation

Incorrect chart

REGULAR PRESCRIPTION — MONTH: APRIL   YEAR 2007

DIGOXIN   liquid   Wrong formulation

WARFARIN   Incorrect area

Dose not specified   CO-CODAMOL   Combination drug

PARACETAMOL   Duplicated drug

CYCLIZINE   Route not specified

GENTAMICIN   Wrong drug/dose

Prescribing | 85

1. Can you think how medication errors are classified? This may help you understand the types of mistakes that can occur and prevent you from making them in the future. See if you can use this as a check list when spotting errors on drug charts.

2. What other errors can you spot on drug charts? If you do spot any thing that you are unsure of, then ensure you speak to the responsible doctor/pharmacist. You may prevent a potential medication error.

Types of medication error	Patients at risk of medication incidents
Wrong patient	Patients who are allergic
Wrong dose, strength or frequency	Children and elderly people
Wrong medicine	Renal and liver dysfunction
Wrong formulation	Patients moving across care settings
Wrong route	Patients cared for outside normal processes
Omitted medicine	

55. Know your abbreviations but do not abbreviate

Medicine is notorious for abbreviations. Drug charts and medications are no exception. Despite the fact that medication names should not be abbreviated, they often are by the hurried doctor. This has previously led to serious medication errors and the death of patients.

Make a list of the abbreviations you have come across and define/write out the drug name in full.

Nakul Patel, Surgeon and Author

Taking it a step further

1. Extend your list to abbreviations that you come across ine medical notes, handover sheets etc. Which acronyms have two or more meanings? Are there any double meanings that are amusing or entertaining? Which ones are potentially dangerous?

2. Carry out an audit looking at numbers of inappropriate abbreviations used on drugs charts (Task 96).

Theme: your peripheral brain – the BNF (*British National Formulary*)

Background

As a doctor you have to remember and recall large amounts of information. You are unlikely to remember all medications, indications, side effects and drug interactions for a patient's drug list. This is why you have the BNF (which is available both as a book and accessible over the internet, or even on mobile phone applications). Prescribing blindly when you don't know the drug is unsafe practice.

Requirements

This theme simply requires a BNF or equivalent for other countries, patients' drug charts plus or minus a willing colleague.

56. Navigating your way through the BNF

This indispensable reference book (or the online version of the book at **www.bnf. org**) will be one of the most useful resources that you will have available to you when you start working. It is usually the first port of call when dealing with medication issues. As a result, if you can master using this resource as a medical student, you would have invested in your own future career.

In the long term, you will have made your life easier and more efficient. In the shorter term, it will prove useful because some medical schools have OSCE stations in which you have to carry out an exercise using the BNF.

However way you look at it, spending some time with your friendly BNF is well worth it. It is no wonder that we have had so many suggestions based around the BNF.

Let's see how well you know the BNF

- How many sections does the BNF have? And how is it divided?
- What are the subsections for each drug?
- What do the appendices cover?
- How to I check for drug interactions?
- What about children?
- How do I check to see what antibiotics can be diluted in saline or dextrose or water?
- Can a pregnant woman take this medication?
- How do I reverse this anticoagulant?
- How do I prescribe a controlled drug, such as morphine?
- My patient is allergic to penicillin. What antibiotic can I prescribe?
- How do you report an adverse drug reaction?
- When do I use the yellow card?

Taking it a step further

With the permission of a doctor on the ward, look through a patient's drug charts and how they are filled in. If there are any drugs that you have not heard of, look them up in the BNF. This will help with knowing how to fill in drug charts and looking up information in the BNF (the BNF can, at first, be a very difficult place to quickly find relevant information and getting used to its format and layout will be helpful). This can be done by yourself or a group of friends who look up one drug each and then explain to the others about what the drug is, its indication, side effects, etc. Working as a group will help with pharmacology and communication skills.

Ravi Agarwal, Medical Student, UK

Look at a set of patient's notes and write down all the drugs they are on from their drug chart. Then go and sit in a quiet area and, next to each drug, write down what each drug is for. After having written this, get a BNF and check you have everything correct and then write down one fact that you didn't already know about the drug from the BNF. This will help you to learn new drug information and revise your existing knowledge of drugs.

Asma Fazlanie, Medical Student, UK

The BNF contains much information; in parts, the text becomes rather microscopic. You are not likely to need to remember all this information. However, as you work on the wards it soon becomes apparent as to which drugs are most commonly prescribed, how they are administered, at what dose and at what times. In addition, common drug interactions and contraindications become apparent.

Looking up medications can be a useful exercise as you will become more familiar with this resource and also building on your foundation of knowledge.

57. Personal BNF

Keep your own personal formulary of regularly used medications. These can be kept on a pocket-size notebook or flashcards (Task 5) or PDA or mobile phone. In this manner you will slowly but steadily build up a list of regularly used medications and will form a good basis for your revision and life as a junior doctor. You might want to structure your formulary according to the BRAInS AIMS mnemonic in the introduction, or other key characteristics of the medication, perhaps including common doses.

When you find yourself bored on the wards, pick a selection of patients and look through their respective drug charts. The drugs listed can then be looked up in the BNF to find out:

(a) what they are and mechanism of action
(b) what their uses are, for this patient and in general
(c) route of administration and suitable doses.

Students can then keep a personal formulary booklet of the drugs they have seen and how then are given in the hope that once they qualify they may feel more comfortable at prescribing the common drugs, and may even remember some doses and routes of admin without having to double-check when on a ward round.

Anneka Rose, Medical Student, UK

58. Peer-based pharmacology learning

Peer-based learning is essential for medical training. Medical students have found this to be engaging and an enjoyable way of learning. This has been found to be one of the most useful methods of studying. (See Section 4 for more information on peer-based learning.)

Learning pharmacology can be made fun with interactive peer-based learning.

This is a 'game' in which two or medical students can play on the ward quietly while waiting for a ward round to start or while waiting for a doctor to teach them, etc.

Basically one student opens a random page of the BNF and names a drug ... the other student must then say as much as they know about the drug, like what class of drugs it is, what dose is usually prescribed, what it is contraindicated in, etc.

If the student does not know then the person with the BNF explains it to them and then the BNF is passed to the next person. The BNF is only passed to the next person after someone gets it wrong.

This helps with memorising drugs and pharmacology and only requires one BNF which is frequently available on all wards.

It's a great way to quietly revise with each other without making too much noise or getting in the way of the nurses.

Asma Fazlanie, Medical Student, UK

This is how a very good friend and I spent the whole of the third year.

In pairs starting at bed number one, regardless of who is looking after the patient, or what the patient has come in for, take the drug chart and starting with the first medication, student number 1 tells student number 2:

~ Indications
~ Mechanisms
~ Adverse effects
~ Contraindications
~ Routes of administration
~ Interactions
~ Related drugs

Keep going around all the different patients and eventually you will be able to understand drugs a bit better.

Do the same for emergency situations ... acute MI, hyperkalaemia, acute asthma, PE.

Sharon Bone, Medical Student, UK

See also:
Building Quizzes, Section 1, Tasks 3–7.

Theme: hidden teachers in pharmacology

Background

Who can teach me pharmacology? Is it the lecturers from your medical school? Or is it the pharmacy department? Well the answer is yes and yes, but there are many more people who can actually teach you. It is a matter of identifying the hidden teachers within your workplace, then utilising your 'cheek and charm' talent to tap into those resources (Section 8). The journey of medicines from production, to prescribing and dispensing requires numerous disciplines, all of which are potential learning opportunities.

Requirements

The identification of an appropriate professional with time to talk and teach.

59. The junior doctor and patient

The 'patient' is a fantastic underused resource. Many patients are so-called expert patients who know about their condition and treatment to a high level.

Find an expert patient on long-term warfarin therapy; he or she may be a good resource to learn about:

- warfarin dosing
- its drug interactions including that with grapefruit and antibiotics
- monitoring INRs (international normalised ratios) and dosing
- recording INRs in the 'yellow book'.

When it came to final year and we were first introduced to prescribing, I found I had paid no attention to drugs that were prescribed on the wards so knew little of doses, sections of the chart to write things in, etc. Therefore when bored, it would be an idea to know the history of a patient and then have a look at their drug chart and try to figure out why a certain drug is being prescribed.

Nkem Okolo, Doctor, UK

Taking it a step further
Junior doctors are a useful but sometimes a rare commodity. Cheek and charm!

60. What would you prescribe?

Pick a patient you have clerked and know well, or think of a scenario that you need to know (asthma, COPD). Write up all the drugs you would prescribe in that situation on the drug chart and then go through it later with the SHO/PRHO.

Emma Short, Medical Student, UK

61. The pharmacist

When on the wards and all the consultants/registrars, etc. seem to have disappeared ... latch on to the pharmacist. Looking at drug charts is all good and well but the pharmacist will be able to tell you about the drug. Follow them and find out why certain drugs are used over others ... how do you get around certain drug idiosyncrasies, how do you administer certain drugs when the charts say the patient is to be 'nil by mouth'? You may be thinking that you could read it all up in the BNF but relating it to the patient and learning it from someone often makes it stick better. Also the pharmacists often know some handy ways to remember drugs.

Thorrmela Vijayaseelan, Medical Student, UK

If you are feeling a little more social then you may wish to go and take a focused drug history from a patient or watch this being done by the pharmacist.

See also
Section 2 for more on taking a history.

62. The nursing staff

Go with some of the nursing staff trained in giving intravenous medications when they are doing their intravenous medication drugs round. This way you can get practice in calculating, drawing up and giving intravenous medications under supervision.

Alison Bradley, Medical Student, UK

During medical school and since as a junior doctor one thing I felt was lacking in our teaching was some very basic skills, such as putting up IV fluids and preparing and giving IV/IM drugs. Although these are taught during the course, we don't often practise them. However, sometimes as a very junior doctor I found myself having to do this, either during emergency situations, or with drugs that nursing staff were not happy to give. While on the wards, I suggest that when bored, medical students ask a nurse if they can observe them putting up IV fluids, to make sure they are confident in how to assemble giving sets. And more importantly, ask if they can assist with the IV drugs round; this is good practice in calculating drug doses in preparation, making up the drug and then giving IV drugs with supervision. It does not take long and these rounds happen regularly throughout the day so when bored on the ward there is nearly always someone about to give IV medication. Not only will doing this provide revision for OSCE exams (where there is often an IV fluids or drugs giving station), but also help prepare medical students for their jobs as junior doctors.

Anna Green, Doctor, UK

63. The pain team

The need for effective pain control is ubiquitous in medicine and permeates the work of all healthcare professionals. If a patient is in pain their recovery will be delayed, they will be unable to maximise the benefit of physiotherapy and occupational therapy exercises, they will be exposed to complications of reduced mobility and their quality of care will be substandard. The bottom line is that you need to become effective in both acute and chronic pain management. So if you have a spare half-hour why not arrange in advance to have a talk with the pain team. This will give you a holistic view of pain management and practical tips on prescribing analgesia (for example, doses and which types of analgesia work well together and which don't) and the role of alternative therapy such as acupuncture.

Alison Bradley, Medical Student, UK

Theme: transition to junior doctor

The transition from medical student to junior doctor always comes quicker than you think. Why not try to take your learning further, such that you begin to start thinking like a junior doctor. Here are two examples to start to get you thinking.

Drug doses

Read through a patient's drug chart. Make sure you understand what each medication is and why it has been prescribed. At medical school, drug dosages are not very important but it will make life easier as a junior doctor if you start to familiarise yourself with the doses commonly used.

Ronan McGinty, Doctor, UK

64. Prescribing cost-effectively

Modern medicine in combination with the increasing number of elderly patients creates a situation where more and more patients due to their multi-morbidity are on many drugs.

This creates interactions, either increasing or decreasing the drug's efficacy, aggravating side effects...

Very often clinicians don't take the time to review adequately the patients' charts regarding their medication; thus it would be a great opportunity for students to learn, on the one hand, how medication is applied and works and, on the other, ultimately reducing the costs of the medications by deleting unnecessary drugs from the patient's treatment. Indeed by discussing each decision with a responsible doctor.

Daniel Jodocy, Medical Student, Austria

65. Insulin and blood sugars

Read through a patient's insulin chart. Observe any changes in the types of insulin or in the dose of insulin given in relation to the patient's BM. If insulin has been prescribed in advance (i.e. based on an expected BM rather than an actual reading), check that the patient's BMs have not become deranged.

Ronan McGinty, Doctor, UK

Further reading

Baker EH, Pryce Roberts AL, Wilde K, Walton H, Suri S, Rull G and Webb AJ (2011). Development of a core drug list towards improving prescribing education and reducing errors in the UK. *British Journal of Clinical Pharmacology* Feb;**71**(2):190–8.

National Coordinating Council for Medication Error Reporting and Prevention: www.nccmerp.org.

National Patient Safety Agency: www.nrls.npsa.nhs.uk/home.

Section 6
BEING CURIOUS

My goal is simple. It is a complete understanding of the universe, why it is as it is and why it exists at all.

Stephen Hawking

Introduction

Somehow I can't believe there are many heights that can't be scaled by a man who knows the secret of making dreams come true. This special secret can be summarized in four C's. They are: curiosity, confidence, courage, and constancy, and the greatest of these is confidence.

Walt Disney

'Knowing about' and 'heard of'

One of the most significant ways of thinking in medical education, and particularly in writing and designing exams, was started by George Miller, who described four different levels on which a student could be examined. At the basic level was the simple 'Know'.

1. 'Know': if they wanted to know if you could take blood safely, examiners might ask about your knowledge of risk, or of what bottles to use. etc. …

2. 'Know how': here they might ask you to describe how you would take blood. …

3. 'Shows': at this stage you might asked to show the examiner how you take blood on a patient or a rubber arm. …

4. 'Does': at this level, the assessors are actually interested in what you do in practice, every day, not just when you are on best behaviour.

Written tests tend to examine the lowest two levels. Most clinical tests examine 'Shows'. Assessing people on what they actually **do** remains a challenge – as soon as they know that they are being watched people tend to 'perform'. You will note that, in some of our tasks, we suggest that you ask colleagues to watch you when you are not expecting them to, e.g. hand washing (Task 47) and manual handling (Task 38), to try to get around this challenge.

101 Things to Do with Spare Moments on the Ward, First Edition. Dason E Evans, Nakul Gamanlal Patel.
© 2012 Dason E Evans and Nakul Gamanlal Patel. Published 2012 by Blackwell Publishing Ltd.

In an easy to read commentary in the *BMJ* (see Further reading), Ed Peile proposed adding another two levels to Miller's pyramid: 'knowing about' and 'heard of' (see diagram). This has a lot of relevance to your time on the wards. As a doctor you will be expected to know a lot, know how to do things (perhaps under supervision) and to be able to perform a wide range of skills competently (show how and do). But, in addition, you will be expected to 'know about' a very wide range of things. You would not expect gynaecologists, for example, to know a lot about colonoscopy, certainly not enough to gain the patient's informed consent, and clearly not enough to be able to perform the procedure. You would, however, expect them to **know** enough **about** colonoscopy to give the patient whom they are referring to the gastroenterologists an overview of the procedure, and answer some of their basic questions.

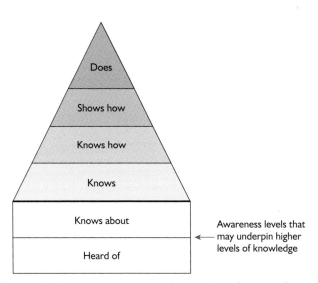

Miller's pyramid of assessable competencies adapted to include levels of awareness. (Reproduced from Peile [2006], with permission from BMJ Publishing Group Ltd.)

Similarly, there may be some things that are so rare, or so unusual or so new, that only a few people know about them in detail. As a doctor, however, you would be expected to have 'heard of' many of these things, so that when one of your patients mentions it you can say 'Yes, I've heard of that, I don't know much about it, tell me what you understand about it, and I know where to look it up to fill in any gaps'. Examples may include gamma knife therapy or percutaneous radiofrequency ablation. For diagnoses, if you have 'heard about' the diagnosis, then you will be able to consider it, even if you need to look it up to be sure. If you have never 'heard about' the diagnosis, you could be in trouble.

Therefore, the point of your time on the wards is not just to gain experience and become knowledgeable about the conditions and skills listed in your core curriculum. One of the main outcomes of your time should also be to gain **experiences** outside the core curriculum, to build up your database of **knows about** and **heard of** so that you will become a wiser and better doctor.

In this section we consider 'knowing about' other professions, including nurses and the confusing variety of other professionals you will see on the wards, knowing about what patients get told, and finding out about and understanding the structure of hospitals and the wider NHS. Within the other sections of this book, you will discover strategies for developing your knowledge about a wide range of procedures, medicines and conditions. If this book had one key message running throughout it, it would be to 'be curious'.

Understanding ('knowing about') other professions

Health professionals work in teams, with different members of the team having different areas of expertise relating to patient care. When the interprofessional team works well together, patient care is optimised. Unfortunately, the different professions tend to have different languages (the word 'care' means very different things to a doctor and a nurse, for example) and often very different world views (a doctor may see a patient's disease progression in terms of chance of cure or haematological markers of progression or patient symptoms, whereas an occupational therapist may focus on what the patient can **do**, particularly with respect to self-care, and how that might change over time). As language tends to be used to define concepts, and as many people tend to assume that everyone else has the same world view as them, these differences in language and world view can lead to considerable conflict, dissonance and inefficient patient care within the interprofessional team.

These challenges have led to a rise in popularity of 'interprofessional learning' – interventions often in the early years of medical school aimed to help students of different professions learn 'with, from and about each other'. It is not unusual for these interventions to be poorly run, resulting in considerable negative feelings within student bodies. If you have been part of a bad 'interprofessional learning' experience, put that aside; this section is about patient care: learning what you need to know in order to work productively with colleagues from other professions to provide excellent patient care.

There are four different aspects of another profession's role that we would recommend that you focus your curiosity on. First, what do they do, what do they not do, what is unique about what they do compared with other professions? This may seem like an easy question, but you will soon discover that different healthcare professions' roles overlap considerably, and this varies between different hospitals and even different departments. Second, what are the internal procedures that each profession has, how are they structured? For example, nursing handover is very different from doctor's handover. Third, what are the differences in use of language? The more you look into this the more fascinated you will become. The term 'clinical skill', for example, means different things to a nurse and a doctor, and covers a fundamentally different concept for speech and language therapists. Fourth and last, consider the world view of each profession. Talk to members of the profession and try to gain an understanding. Examples of areas to explore include: What is patient care about for a nurse? What would be a success in terms of a good patient outcome? What would be a failure? These four areas (you can probably add more, if you like) will help you gain an understanding of what each of the other professions is actually 'about' and that understanding will make working with them much easier and more productive in the years to come.

> **Useful areas of exploration to gain an understanding of other professions**
> 1. What do they do?
> 2. What internal procedures do they have?
> 3. What are the differences in use of language?
> 4. What world view do they have?

If you are still cynical about anything with the word 'interprofessional' in the title, remember that the suggestions in this section are principally written by students, reflecting **things** that they have found useful in helping them understand the other professions. They clearly thought that these **things to do** were useful and productive. Why not give it a go?

Summary

Having a broad knowledge of medical practice is an essential foundation to being a doctor, and we hope that this section will encourage you to spend time exploring areas outside your core curriculum. We have deliberately clustered interprofessional learning within this section, because we believe that it is not something special or different; understanding other professions is simply another area of medicine that you will need to know about in order to provide excellent patient care as a doctor.

We hope that you will realise that, although this section focuses on **heard of**, **know about** and **understanding other professions**, these themes run through many of the other sections of the book. When gaining anatomy teaching in the interventional radiology department, for example Task 83, you are likely to see some unusual procedures, which will make you wiser ('know about'). Similarly, when shadowing the thrombolysis nurse practitioner or the echo operators (Section 3) make sure that you learn about these other professions, as well as about the procedures that you are observing.

Theme: a doctor's best friend: the nurse

Background

Nurses are a great source to learn from; many of them have been working in the hospital for decades and will have picked up many useful day-to-day tips and tricks for tasks that you as a junior will be required to carry out. As someone so fresh into the working environment, they are a cohort that can teach you many basic skills, introduce you to patients with rare disorders and take off certain job responsibilities, which in turn makes your life a lot less stressful. Of course, this is even more relevant for the medical student.

Have you ever wondered how your consultant knows how you have been performing without ever being around? Do they have extraterrestrial powers? Or big brother cameras on the ward? No, but many consultants have a good relationship with the nursing staff and many senior nurses may have known your consultants from when they were junior doctors. So if you impress the nurses, you surely will be doing yourself a favour when they inform your consultants.

You will be working with nurses for the rest of your career: Understanding what they do (and don't do) and what their world view is will be incredibly useful to you for the rest of your life.

Requirements

The tasks below require willing nursing staff of varying specialist areas who are happy to let you observe, help and talk to them.

66. Shadow a nurse

Nurses are an excellent source of knowledge and simply shadowing them will lead to a better understanding of their role and better team work.

Nurse specialists are an excellent source of knowledge and information. Ask to spend the morning with, or arrange a 30-minute talk with, a specialist nurse. Not only will you gain a better appreciation of their role but you will also see what information they give to their patients and how they communicate this information to their patients. This will not only help your communication skills but will also enhance your patient management plans in the future as you will know when to involve nurse specialists early in your patient's care.

Alison Bradley, Medical Student, UK

Taking it a step further

Taking it a step further, you can arrange to meet one of the many nurse specialists and learn exactly what she or he does. You will soon realise that there is much overlap between your roles. You may also gain some practical skills as shown in the next task.

Make a list of all the types of nurse specialists you know and see if they are present at your hospital.

67. Handover

You will always find doctors and nurses within the hospital regardless of the time of day or night. With the implementation of the European Working Time Directive (EWTD), there has been an increase in the number of shifts and a resultant increase in the number of handovers. The information passed at handover is necessary to ensure good continuity of care.

Useful information is passed over during handover between the various nursing shifts. If medical students asked to be present during report they will get to know what is required for each patient and could volunteer to help carry out some of these procedures/tasks.

Klaudine Simpson, Senior Clinical Skills Tutor, UK

Taking it a step further

The quality of handovers can be poor with the lack of essential information being passed on. A good example is when there is a critically unwell patient. You could carry out your own analysis of how good you rate different handovers. What is done well and what can be improved upon? Would a computerised system be better? Is there a leader or coordinator? Is there opportunity for questions?

You could also compare handovers between different healthcare professionals such as doctors, nurses, physiotherapists and nurses.

You could also compare handovers between different grades of doctors: foundation doctors, senior house officers, registrars and consultants?

Meera Patel, Dentist and Author, UK

Make cups of tea for the nurses and sit down with them for a while — they usually have some words of wisdom for young doctors and a few good stories to tell!

Elizabeth Tissingh, Foundation Year 1 Doctor, UK

68. Friend or foe — you choose

In every profession, you can meet some 'challenging personalities' and the nursing profession (and, indeed medical profession) is no exception. Remember to show respect and in turn you will gain it. A poor relationship with nurses as a new doctor will have a negative impact on patient care and can cause additional pressure to an already hectic start as a junior.

Be friendly and approachable with the nurses and maintain a professional relationship, so that you are taken seriously. This is a tricky skill to attain and watching your seniors can be a good place to start learning this skill. You will find that some of your colleagues do have a healthy relationship whereas, others do not — you can learn from both groups.

Make friends with the nurses — take 5 minutes out of your time to make small talk with the nurses. They can help you more than you could imagine — or they could make your life hell. PICK THE FORMER!

Ziena Abdullah, Medical Student, UK

If you're bored and think there's nothing to do, then why not talk to the nursing staff on the ward. If you take the time to get to know them both as professionals and as people then you'll not only get to learn more about what everyone else does, but you'll also make friends with them. That way, if something interesting crops up then they'll let you know. Helping empty bedpans and stripping a bed might not seem like your idea of fun but it could end up paying for itself when the nurse you helped tells you about the patient with the rare condition on the next ward along.

Simon Stallworthy, Medical Student, UK

If you are sitting on the ward doing nothing, ask the nurses if there is anything you can do. Let them know that you are eager to do anything and are trained in most investigative techniques. By doing this you will learn and get the opportunity to do things like: venepuncture, insertion of Venflons, setting up an IV bag or ECGs. These are all jobs that nurses routinely do and if they know that you are eager to help then you can gain lots of valuable clinical experience.

Donna Pilkington, Medical Student, UK

Taking it a step further

Observe which junior doctors have better professional relationships with the nurses. How do they manage this? Compare their behaviour and attitudes to those juniors who tend to find their nursing colleagues more challenging.

Theme: who are the players?

Background

Who works on the ward? The patient journey is made up of various direct and indirect interactions with healthcare professionals and allied supporting staff other than doctors and nurses. It is often easy to dismiss the essential roles of others and assume that only doctors and nurse work on the ward.

Nevertheless, the safe admission, inpatient stay, investigations, rehabilitation and discharge of patients require a complex interaction of various 'players'. Much like a sports team, each player has a vital role. In order for the team to perform well each of the players needs to perform their individual parts well. A hospital team is made up of a much more complex group and is subdivided into small teams. To appreciate what each of the players do we first need to know whom they are.

There is also a bigger picture; the different players sit within a wider hospital structure, which sits within an even wider healthcare context including primary care, funding bodies, quality enhancement bodies and, of course, medical schools. Patients navigate a complex pathway through all this complexity, and these pathways are caught, described and documented.

Requirements

The requirements for the tasks below are the specific people who work in the hospital: healthcare professionals or allied supporting staff. You can gain much from either shadowing them or simply talking to them. The former will be much better because it will form a deeper form of learning taking you up Miller's pyramid.

Some of the tasks require a fellow medical student who is equally bored on the ward.

---

69. Get to know the other teams!

If you are on the ward, find out how it is organised. If there is a secretary who plans rounds, visits, special examinations, ask her/him to warn you if there is a patient undergoing special examinations like heart catheterisation, or IVP, or special physiotherapy, occupational

---

therapy, group therapy, etc. Ask the patient and physician or therapist if you can join this.

Germaine Leunissen, Doctor and Teacher, The Netherlands

70. Getting to know the hospital vampires

This section had many submissions, perhaps because it is readily examined or these are core skills that are required from the first day as a junior doctor. The important thing here is to see how different approaches can be used to the same task of learning to take bloods or placing an intravenous cannula.

If you have some time on your hands go to the haematology day unit and spend some time with the nurses there; you can spend as much or as little time as you want but there are always patients who need cannulas and bloods done. The nurses are really experienced and so are really good at teaching how to put cannulas in and are patient with you as they do not often have many students; the patients are also normally used to having cannulas put in so are very kind if you have to do it more than once. In addition to the hands-on stuff you get to write out the blood forms, post them in the chute (very useful for becoming an F1), looking in notes and seeing what blood tests need to be performed with different types of treatment ... rather than everything ... with the interpretation of the results being essential (also good practice).

Note that it is always nice to ask the nurses if it is right to turn up at some point; they also like chocolate!

Linzi Arkus, Medical Student, UK

See also submissions for Task 44 onward.

Taking it a step further
You can apply this to more than just cannulas and can extend your skill mix to include learning how to perform echocardiograms or take arterial blood gases.

As long as the ward is not deadly quiet, take a look around ... there may be staff other than doctors around who can be invaluable in terms of providing knowledge. There maybe phlebotomists, echo operators and specialists. Ask kindly if you can tag along for a while and, provided they let you, you can gain knowledge on a multitude of things ... whether it be taking blood, important findings on echo, etc. ... .

Laura Geddes, Medical Student, UK

When you have perfected taking bloods you can look at the possible anatomical sites available to take blood in both an elective and emergency setting. You could compare the peripheral and central venous access sites and possible complications of both. This would help you learn your anatomy, apply it to a clinical setting and understand the possible complications of your procedure.

Meera Patel, Dentist and Author, UK

If you have spare time during the day with nothing to do, you can go to the radiology department and ask for some teaching. They enjoy teaching students and I felt there was not enough radiology teaching in our course anyway, so it's a good chance for some small group teaching.

Second idea is similar but go to bloods/phlebotomy department and ask to observe and then take blood. If you go down and see them, book a clinic. Good for third years.

Last idea: go find an endoscopy clinic if you have a free afternoon. Good teaching on anatomy and helpful if you are not on a gastro firm.

Odelia Amit, Medical Student, UK

71. Uniform recognition

There are many uniforms in the hospital. Recognising who wears which uniform is the first step in getting to appreciate who each member of the team is.

If you're hanging around waiting for a ward round to start, try to work out what the roles of all the other health professionals who are wandering around are. You get to recognise the various different uniforms of different professions and see what they do. Ask someone if you're not sure. After a while you get a much better idea of all-round patient care and also know who to ask about various different aspects of it when you get stuck.

Jennifer Pennekett, Medical Student, UK

72. The multidisciplinary team and clinical effectiveness

Understanding the **language** that different members of the multidisciplinary team (MDT) speak will go a long way in your career. A useful place to see them all interact is the clinical effectiveness meeting.

If you are on placement and you hear of a clinical effectiveness meeting coming up, try to go along. At these meetings the multidisciplinary team discuss issues arising in the work place. As a student you might think why should you go along but it is good to gain insight into issues that prevent the MDT from working well together. If you learn what doctors are doing that annoys other members of the team and vice versa, you will begin your working life with an insight into how you can avoid interdisciplinary tension and maximise your working relationship within the MDT.

Alison Bradley, Medical Student, UK

73. Radiology requests

As junior doctors, your consultant may ask you to request umpteen plain radiographs, and CT and MRI scans. Why are so many of them rejected by the radiologist? A better understanding of what light an investigation throws on the clinical question will lead you to give more appropriate requests with the relevant succinct details on the request form. You will, in turn, have your request performed sooner with less interrogation.

This was again a high submissions topic and we agree that time spent performing these tasks will be most beneficial to your working life.

When you start working you will find yourself requesting numerous scans for your patients as part of your busy workload. Therefore, as a student, if you find yourself with a spare morning or afternoon why not go to the radiology department and see a few MR, CT, CTPA scans, etc. being done. You can learn so much from doing this including: what each investigation will/will not show, how to discern normal anatomy from positive findings on scans, and indications and contraindications for these scans. You will also pick up handy tips on how to fill out request forms properly so that, when you are working as a busy junior doctor, you will be less likely to find your requests being rejected due to lack of relevant clinical information on the request form. Also if you see these scans, you will be better equipped to explain to your patient what is involved from their point of view and in a language they will understand.

Alison Bradley, Medical Student, UK

Take it a step further
Time spent at the CT scanner will also allow you to understand how the procedure is carried out and thus help when patients ask about what the investigation entails.

I had half a day free recently and wandered down to the radiology department to see if I was able to watch some CT scans being performed. The radiologists were only to happy to let me watch and also talk through the kinds of things they were looking for and what they might suggest, so I learnt a great deal about interpreting CT scans which I had previously found a bit difficult. Having never seen a CT scanner before it was also very interesting to see the process of a CT being taken and I thought it was important for me to know the process so as to be able to explain to patients exactly what was going to happen to them when sent for a CT scan.

Jennifer Pennekett, Medical Student, UK

If you have a spare half-hour it would be a good idea to call into the radiology department and find out when patients are having barium meal studies performed. It is good to see exactly what this investigation involves as you will gain a better appreciation of which patients are/are not suitable for this investigation. Also if you see this investigation being performed yourself, it will be easier to explain the procedure to your patients in a way they will better understand. Furthermore as a medical student you will see exactly what this investigation does and does not show in terms of assisting in making a diagnosis.

Alison Bradley, Medical Student, UK

74. The bigger picture

In the introduction we mentioned the jungle that is the health service, the complex interactions between different 'stakeholders' and the patient pathways that facilitate easy passage between them. Endless reforms and restructuring make the situation even more difficult to understand.

Spend some time with colleagues considering the structure of the hospital that you are in, including its lines of management, and consider how this fits into the NHS. How does the hospital get its money? How is it distributed? Who manages the nurses? Who manages the doctors? How does an outpatient appointment get paid for? Write down as many questions as you can think of, and search out the answers.

Dason Evans, Doctor and Author

Theme: communication

Section 2 covers learning clinical communication; within this theme we highlight what can be learnt from communication – written, electronic, and web based, with an emphasis on 'knowing about'. This section overlaps with Section 2 and also with some of Section 1.

75. What do patients get told?

Leaflets are a good source of information when written in layman language and illustrated with diagrams in a language that the patient understands. It is also something concrete that the patient can refer to when they want to check something after their consultation, and it helps fill the large gap between what the clinician believes they have explained and what the patient recalls being told.

Medical students can go to the endoscopy department of a hospital and ask for patient information leaflets about colonoscopy, flexible sigmoidoscopy, OGD, etc. This will help you to understand these procedures better and they will be written in simple language (as they are intended for patients) and so will help with 'informed consent' OSCE stations. It is also useful, after gaining permission from the doctor and the patient, to observe these procedures.

Ravi Agarwal, Medical Student, UK

Taking it a step further

'We'll give you a leaflet, Mrs Brown ...'

Medical students are encouraged to think about providing patient information in alternative formats (written, website, etc.). But giving someone printed information can become an easy option that may not help the patient as much as we might imagine:

1. Find a patient who is happy for you to spend a little time with them. Try to choose someone who may not find it straightforward to use typical information leaflets. Perhaps they don't have English as a first language, they have vision problems or reading difficulties (although people often hide this), they are physically unable to hold an information sheet (e.g. patients with rheumatoid arthritis), or they have a learning disability.

If you can't find a patient like this, it doesn't matter. Whatever they tell you will help you!

2. Ask what information they have been given about their condition (other than verbally, from a health professional). If possible, take a look. In what form was it given? How helpful (or not) was it, and why?

3. After you've thanked the patient, use what you have learned. If the patient has had no information and would like some, what would best meet their needs? (Check with nursing staff before you offer information.) Or if the patient was given a fantastic leaflet that really helped them understand, say, type 2 diabetes, ask yourself: suppose this patient spoke only Tamil? Or was partially sighted or totally blind? What would be available to help them?

4. Now look for sources of patient information. What is available on the ward, or in the clinic? If it's all printed and in English, which is most likely, you'll need to look further afield. Who is responsible for patient information in your Trust? (This varies widely.) Ask at the nurses' station, look on the Trust intranet or call the switchboard. There may be a patient information centre; PALS might be a good source; or try the communications office. Be prepared to trek round the hospital, and don't forget the internet.

5. You may, or may not, find what you want. Most hospitals will not have stockpiles of, say, audiotapes in Gujarati about cutting your risk

of heart disease. (This isn't necessarily through lack of thought; cost is inevitably a factor.) The point is to think about what a patient's communication needs might be, how you could address them ... and why it's good practice to think before telling a patient 'We'll give you a leaflet'!

Anna Jenkins, Medical Student, UK

76. Intranet

The intranet site is another useful site of communication and usually contains useful information. Many hospital Trusts have antibiotic guidelines, treatment of medical emergencies, access to the BNF and other useful links.

Look at the Trust's intranet site for chaplaincy and inform yourself about the range of chaplaincy available in the Trust so that you can pass that information on to your patients as required.

The Revd Peter Cowell, Chaplain, UK

Taking it a step further
We are living in an age of information overload with the media — newspapers, magazines, radio, television and the internet! There are many sources that may not be completely accurate. Why don't you produce some accurate patient information and see if you can produce material for the Trust in any media described.

Gaman Patel, Businessman, UK

References/further reading

Miller's pyramid is discussed well in most medical education books, and online in a range of sources.
Peile E (2006). Knowing and knowing about. *BMJ* **332**:645.
Freeth D (2007) *Interprofessional Education*. Edinburgh: ASME – Association for the Student of Medical Education.

Section 7
DATA INTERPRETATION

Although we often hear that data speak for themselves, their voices can be soft and sly.
Stephen M Stigler

Introduction

Being a doctor in many ways resembles being a detective, working out what might be wrong, looking for clues, ordering appropriate investigations and then interpreting the data in the clinical context to formulate an appropriate diagnosis. It is only at this stage that you are able to initiate appropriate treatments for your patient.

Interpreting data is an essential skill for a doctor. It is likely to be tested throughout your medical studies including in Objective Structured Clinical Examinations (OCSEs). The best way to learn this skill is first to recognise what is normal and then practice, practice, practice!

Using real patient data (i.e. radiographs, ECGs and drug charts of ward patients) is an excellent way to learn. If you can begin to do this while at medical school, you are half-way on the way to being able to do it when you are the person looking after the patient.

There are many times when data are interpreted incorrectly, resulting in the diagnosis being wrong, which can lead to the administration of incorrect treatment and potentially patient harm. This goes against your first duty of care: 'do no harm!'.

Another reason to become very slick at interpreting data accurately is because it is **always** incorporated in verbal and practical examinations at undergraduate level.

It is also vital to understand that tests can be adjuncts to confirm or refute a clinical diagnosis. Thus, despite the fact that some of our examples are taken outside the clinical context, it is prudent to relate the test result to the patient. Occasionally, an unexpected result may be secondary to an error and it is important to consider repeating it, (such as an ECG taken with the leads incorrectly placed on the patient).

Interpretation of test results requires knowledge of 'what is normal'. It is therefore important to have a clear understanding of what is normal and what is abnormal. This may not be as easy as it seems – a 50% rise in one of the liver enzymes above normal has a very different level of significance from a 50% rise in plasma potassium levels.

In this section we look at some favourite data interpretation topics covered in ward rounds and examinations.

---

101 Things to Do with Spare Moments on the Ward, First Edition. Dason E Evans, Nakul Gamanlal Patel.
© 2012 Dason E Evans and Nakul Gamanlal Patel. Published 2012 by Blackwell Publishing Ltd.

Theme: patient notes

Background

Patient notes are an essential part of patient care. These include the written notes, laboratory results, clinical photographs and radiographic imaging. With improvements in technology many more resources are IT based, including patient records. You may have also realised that the old light boxes on the walls are almost an antique feature with transfer of imaging on to computer-based systems.

Nevertheless, patient records are legal documents about patient care and it is important to remember that each page in the patient's notes should contain the patient's name and unique identifier. When you chart an entry into the notes you should also write your name, designation, contact number, date and time.

Requirements

The requirements for this section include the patient's notes whether on computer or paper.

77. Knowing what is normal

What is normal? In statistics, the normal distribution, also known as the Gaussian curve, is a continuous probability distribution that describes data that cluster around an average. It forms a bell-shaped curve of what is supposed to be considered 'normal'.

In medicine it is especially important to establish what is normal in order to appreciate pathology. The more times you examine something normal, the easier it will be for you to recognise when things are not right.

Learn normal value for tests so when reading through the notes — the written values included will make sense to you.

Ruth Bird, Medical Student, UK

Feel like a spare wheel?
As a medical student, there will be many a time when you feel in the way. You will not be the only one who has experienced this. However, do not let this dishearten you; instead take advantage of this situation.

Look at X-rays or blood test results of people recently admitted through A&E or who are on the ward.

Try to figure out what the diagnosis is and what your management would be. Only look at the notes when you can get no further on your own.

Elizabeth Tissingh, FY1 Doctor, UK

Ask to see some patients' notes — check with the ward clerk or nurse it's ok to take them and don't leave the ward — tell them exactly where you'll be with the notes. Read through the notes and write down anything you don't understand. Ideally do this with a partner and test one another's knowledge on the particular subject. If there's a computer nearby, use that to look up any unfamiliar terms.

Laura Kendal and Ruth Bird, Medical Students, UK

78. Clinical governance

Clinical governance was introduced to improve the quality of healthcare, manage risk and ensure continuing professional development. It is composed of eight building blocks:

1. **G**reatest health care practice (implementation of best practice)

2. **O**penness and accountability

3. **V**ery happy patients (patient satisfaction)

4. **E**very year: monitor and feedback

5. **R**isk management

6. **A**udit and peer review (see below)

7. **C**ontinuing professional development

8. **E**xcellent professional performance

This can easily be remembered by the mnemonic, GOVERnAnCE (ignore the 'n'). (Section 1, Task 1 for more on mnemonics.)

Audit is a small part of clinical governance and is simply a method of systematically checking the quality of a health service given to patients. It is a great way of improving practice.

It is also something that you will be a part of once you become a doctor, so why not start early. It will look good on your CV and help you in familiarise yourself with the processes involved.

The illustration below shows the various components to the audit cycle. The most important of which is 'repeat audit' such that you are able to close the audit cycle to show whether your intervention has had any impact on the quality of the service.

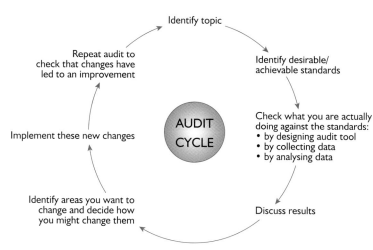

From Patel M, Patel N. (2007) Dental public health: a primer. Radcliffe Oxford with permission.

Relevance of investigations

~ Pick a random set of patient notes (paper or electronic).

~ Have a read through the current admission.

~ Note down all investigations in chronological order and rate the value or appropriateness of the investigation. If you felt the investigation was inappropriate, why do you think it was ordered? Were there investigations that you think were omitted or performed late?

~ What factors influence our decision to order or perform an investigation?

~ Are results always reviewed?

~ How could the system be improved?

~ Should we be accountable for investigations we perform or order?

Consider how this exercise would influence your behaviour.

Andy Wearn, Clinical Senior Lecturer, New Zealand

Taking it further

Get involved with audit, Task 96.

Find out the difference between audit and research; it is a common question at interviews.

79. Efficiency defines your competency

Efficiency is intelligent laziness.

David Dunham

When working in the hospital you soon realise that patient notes are the most poorly organised records of patient care. There are lots of lessons to be learnt.

As a house officer, efficiency defines your competency! Mastering this early on in your career helps you to preserve your sanity and that of the rest of the team! When I followed the consultants through ward rounds, I got frustrated if things were not in order. For example, when I was a house officer in GI medicine, I was always asked about the results of liver screen, the ultrasound report and the endoscopy findings on almost every patient. My SHO and I therefore at our free time developed a concise liver screen results form on one page completed with Maddrey's score and Child-Pugh score. Needless to say, my consultants love it and my life has been easier since!

There is always something in the ward that you could improve on. Look around and start making your life easier. Start a serial blood results form if there isn't one. Make your own proforma and get your seniors to look through it.

Saw Sian Khoo, Doctor, Malaysia

Keep the patients' record books up to date, with all details and progressions, i.e. ward movements, outpatient, etc.

Indrajith Kowarthanan, Medical Student, UK

Another important skill includes making sense of large-volume notes and being able to summarise them all in a few minutes.

During lull periods, or when you are waiting for a doctor to arrive, ask staff members to recommend a patient whose notes you can read.

You can do this for a patient who will be seen next and then you can practise summarising to the consultant or doctor before the patient is seen, or simply to learn more about the condition from the notes, e.g. how it presented, the investigations required, etc. for this particular patient. Any questions can then be immediately addressed by the doctors when they arrive.

Canh Van On, Medical Student, UK

Theme: patient ECGs (Electrocardiogram)

Background

ECG stands for electrocardiogram and gives a trace that reflects the electrical activity of the heart over time. This is captured by externally placed skin electrodes. It is a basic test that is used routinely and as a result you must know about these in detail. Many medical students struggle at first in the skills of recording and interpreting them, but the way to learn is practice, practice and more practice. Below are some ideas for getting to grips and mastering ECGs; try them out.

Learning to record an electrocardiogram

Task 43.

80. Practice, practice, practice

There are numerous books that one can use while learning the theory and also practising; however, the real test is when these can be applied in clinical practice. Is this patient with chest pain having an STEMI (ST-elevation myocardial infarction)? Because this is the time in which your management plan is directly related to this investigation.

ECG practice: most patients (particularly adult general medical/surgical and care of the elderly) have ECGs on admission (and, if not, have old ECGs at the back of their notes). Find a friend and analyse and present these ECGs to each other. Sadly it's a skill that disappears if you don't use it, and as a medical student this is one of the best ways to keep it fresh in your mind!

Sarah Perkin, Medical Student, UK

As a medical student, I've had difficulty in reading ECGs. Take a set of patient notes and there should be an ECG — especially if they're a cardiac patient or they have come in via A&E. Take time to familiarise yourself with it. Go through the various points you have either been taught or read and go through the motions, i.e. correct patient, dates, if performed properly, rhythm, rate and axis, making sure the amplitude and direction of the waves are within correct limits; timing between intervals is not too long or short and finally you can compare it to a previous ECG. You can then present your findings to a doctor if around. The correct finding is usually written on the top of the ECG paper and the rate on the ECG itself! This provides good practice for the data interpretation exam!

Laura Geddes, Medical Student, UK

On every ward there is a trolley with patient notes and radiographs in it. With the permission of a doctor on that ward, you can look through a patient's chest X-rays, abdominal X-rays, head CTs, ECGs, etc. with other students in a systematic way and try to come up with a diagnosis. This can be done in three ways:

(1) by yourself
(2) as a group of students discussing it together
(3) as a group of students thinking about it in their minds and at the end seeing which student came up with the correct diagnosis

You can then check if the diagnosis is correct by looking through the patient's notes. If you come across a particular radiograph or ECG which none of the students can interpret or come up with a diagnosis you can either ask a doctor to go through it with you or read up on it.

Once you become confident at interpreting simple radiographs/ECGs you can ask one of the doctors if there is a radiograph/ECG which is very difficult to interpret and try to make sense of it.

This is useful preparation for radiology data interpretation/OSCE questions.

You can also follow patients up as they have new radiographs/ECGs carried out, interpret them and ask a doctor if you can present your findings to the consultant at the next ward round. This will:

(1) help interpretation skills
(2) build confidence talking about radiographs to your seniors (in an exam you may need to interpret a radiograph to an examiner)
(3) get you noticed if done well!

Ravi Agarwal, Medical Student, UK

81. Pattern recognition

You will soon realise that, like lots of things in medicine, there are patterns which, once you recognise, you will be able to diagnose. You should learn the patterns such as 'WiLLiaM MaRRoW' and eventually try to work out why in bundle-branch blocks you see these patterns. Why do signs of right heart strain signify a pulmonary embolism?

Currently, I am in the cardiology ward of Whipps Cross University Hospital and there are just so many ECGs (it is everywhere!). There are ECGs printed out every day for each patient and they will be filed along with the obs chart, fluid chart, etc. There are monitors with real-time ECGs as well. There is a whole file of ECGs for discharged patients, kept in doctors' room.

So far in my second week, whenever I am bored in the ward, I will be randomly picking one ECG and go through it with my house officers.

I found it very useful in interpreting ECGs and understanding the patient better. The house officers have been very kind to enlighten me on many aspects of ECGs.

ECGs in books such as ECGs Made Easy are never really the same as in real-life ECGs printed from a patient, since there are often multiple problems with one patient's heart. One example is S1Q3T3 for pulmonary embolism, which, according to my consultant, is very rare and not worth looking for. Another example is bundle-branch block. WiLLiaM MaRRoW is very useful; however, some patients' ECGs are never as explicit as explained using WiLLiaM MaRRoW (especially partial block). Students may come across ECGs with no clear W/M on V1/V6, yet a cardiologist will be able to say confidently that the patient does have BBB.

Hopefully, I will be able to interpret more ECGs in my remaining weeks with the cardiology team in Whipps. Just one last thing, ECG is printed for each patient admitted into the hospital, hence students don't have to be in a cardiology ward to have access to it.

Wee Fu Gan, Medical Student, UK

Theme: imaging

Background

The imaging department is one of the most utilised departments within any hospital, with continually improving technologies. Techniques recreate images of parts of the human body to reveal the patient's anatomy and physiology.

It incorporates plain radiographic imaging, magnetic resonance imaging (MRI), nuclear medicine, photoacoustic imaging, breast thermography, tomography and ultrasonography.

As you can see there is a lot more to the imaging department than chest radiographs.

One word of warning: some clinicians feel very strongly that an X-ray image should be called a 'radiograph', because an 'X-ray' is technically a type of electro-magnetic radiation, rather than the image. You will see that we, and most of the people submitting ideas for this book, use the terms rather interchangeably.

Requirements

There are many books on learning how to interpret radiographs, but the best way is to see radiographs for real patients; below are some examples of how you can do so.

82. Utilise technology

You will find that many hospitals have now moved to an electronic system that may require a password. You may have to find a friendly doctor to log you on to the system.

It's simple but very useful.

If you are at a hospital where X-rays are done electronically, rather than printed out; you can spend as much or as little time as you like doing this.

Just simply sit down at the ward computer and go through all the X-rays taken that day and get a feel for looking at them (it doesn't matter if you have not seen the person before).

In 30 min you will probably be able to look at around 30 different X-rays. You might not know exactly what you are looking at but after you have looked at 30 chest X-rays you can begin to get a feel for what is normal and what is abnormal, which is the most important step in looking at X-rays.

It is even better if you do it in groups of two or three as you can pool resources and ideas of your friends.

Michael Magro, Medical Student, UK

Spend time interpreting radiographs/CT/MR films. Although it may be harder for students nowadays to get to see chest radiographs (and interpret them, of course) as all imaging is now in the computer network in most hospitals, ask a doctor to log on to the network for you to access the patient's imaging results.

Wei Yang Low, Medical Student, UK

If the hospital has a central database with X-rays, CT and MR scans uploaded on it and the student has access to it, then going through the radiology and labs of patients on the ward is a good learning opportunity, particularly if a clinician is available to teach. This can be for as little or as long as wished, depending on the time available.

Sarah Onida, Medical Student, UK

Go through the ward chest X-rays, present them to each other as you would do on a ward round. Then try to come up with a management plan based on the finding.

Emma Short, Medical Student, UK

83. Imaging and the other professions

There are many people within the hospital who may be able to help you interpret imaging apart from doctors. A trip down to radiology and spending some time with the radiographer may be helpful, because this will enable you to also see how they take a CT scan. Working with physiotherapists may help you see patients' clinical and radiographic features. For example, basal collapse on a postoperative patient may be found clinically, confirmed by radiology, improved with chest physiotherapy and finally confirmed on a repeat chest radiograph.

When there's no one around from your team, there's always plenty of other departments in the hospital, often without medical students. The X-ray department is a particularly good one to visit, as being able to interpret any kind of scans is a valuable skill. All X-ray departments I have visited so far have been more than willing to let us sit (with patient consent) to watch CT scans while describing what you're seeing on screen. Those willing to teach have often taken us through CTs, MRIs and chest/abdo radiographs at any level – from most basic to rare findings and how to spot them. The same applies to many other departments – cardiac outpatients is another good one for practising placing ECG leads and reading the outputs. No need to wait around for someone to tell you to go to these places.

Fenella Beynon, Medical Student, UK

Getting patients X-rays, CT scans, etc. on the ward and having a look through them on the ward to better understand them and learn from repeated exposure to such radiology. This task takes minimal time and can be stopped very quickly if the Dr/student has to take on another task. This makes it very versatile. If done with other members of staff and other suitable professions, it can be a fun way of sharing ideas and looking at things from different perspectives.

Asheesh Bharti, Medical Student, UK

Going to the radiology department is really useful and really interesting. The radiologists and radiographers do not usually mind and are keen to help, and you can get some teaching (especially anatomy teaching) out of it at the same time. It's also a good opportunity to follow up on a patient you may have clerked and look at the investigations they need. There's lots to see and do too: X-rays, CTs, MRIs, ERCPs, etc. and they might let you put in cannulas for patients that need contrast.

Charity Santeng, Medical Student, UK

84. Self-test

Open up the computer system and pull up scans, either of your own patients or someone else's and, before looking at the scan report, try to write your own/make a spot diagnosis. You can then decide what tests you would order next if you were the treating physician. This is a really good way to get used to looking at scans and presenting (find a friend!). You might also get a prior look at an X-ray your consultant wants you to analyse on ward round, and you'll sound extra clever if you've already had a chance to formulate what you think is going on.

Sarah Perkin, Medical Student, UK

When I am bored and all the junior Drs are otherwise busy, I look for where all the X-rays and scans are stored. Grab a handful and then spend any given amount of time trying to interpret them, and comparing my judgement with the actual report.

Omar Chehab, Medical Student, UK

The medical student should go to the notes trolley and pick up individual patient X-rays. He/she should then present them as if in the exam and then check the report to make sure the diagnosis was correct.

Ziena Abdullah, Medical Student, UK

See also
Task 4 onwards.

85. The secret folder

I recently discovered that most radiology departments keep folders full of teaching films for staff development, training and college examinations, yet never inform students about these gems. Go to the department, suss out a friendly member of staff and ask to see these folders which are often housed away in a dark corner somewhere or even electronically if the dept are computer competent. I have seen all sorts of interesting films this way which have included embedded bullets and uncommon diseases. Hope this helps

Christopher Thexton, Medical Student, UK

We would also like to acknowledge Amanda Jewison and Donna Pilkington for submitting a very similar idea.

Reference

Patel M, Patel N (2007). *Dental Public Health: A primer*. Oxford: Radcliffe.

Section 8
GETTING TEACHING

When the student is ready, the master appears.

Buddhist proverb

Introduction

Some students seem to get lots of teaching on the wards, and others don't. There are three main factors involved. The first is building the right reputation – being recognised as the student who is keen and interested; second, you need the right skills and attitudes when in a situation where teaching could take place ('cheek and charm', 'giving it a go'); and third, a commitment to searching out opportunities for learning. This whole book is about putting you in charge of your learning and teaching, and you may have noticed that these three themes weave like three threads throughout the book, and are embedded within many of the submissions.

This section is, therefore, a relatively short one, not because it is unimportant, but rather because we wanted to pull together these threads in one place, to highlight them.

In the first part of this section we cluster some submissions about motivating others to teach you, and in the second part we cross-reference a lot with the rest of the book, highlighting different people and places where you can find good teaching.

A word on rejection: we all know that an enthusiastic, passionate teacher can motivate us, and fill us with interest for their topic. Unfortunately the opposite is also true. If you ask someone for teaching and they are rude and abrupt, this can seem really devastating, particularly if you found it an effort to gain the courage to ask them in the first place. Don't be deterred; read the section on motivating yourself (Section 9) and try again. Perhaps that clinician was having a tough day, or maybe they are just generally unpleasant; either way, if they are unhappy that a medical student wants to learn, that isn't your problem!

Theme: motivating people to teach you

Background

The unfair truth is that keen students, who do lots, tend to get spotted and offered more opportunities, whereas students who don't appear so motivated tend to get left on the sidelines.

101 Things to Do with Spare Moments on the Ward, First Edition. Dason E Evans, Nakul Gamanlal Patel. © 2012 Dason E Evans and Nakul Gamanlal Patel. Published 2012 by Blackwell Publishing Ltd.

A fourth year student sat in with one of the authors (DE) recently in the sexual health clinic. Sexual health is a nice specialty for students – there are a limited number of common diagnoses and only a handful of commonly used medications. The skills required to take a sexual history can be challenging, but as someone who is 'only a student' you have permission to get it wrong and you also have the luxury of someone experienced enough supervising you to rescue you if things get tricky. All in all, students who prepare a little beforehand and engage can be given quite a lot of responsibility, and learn lots that will be useful outside sexual health.

This student was bored. He hadn't read anything about sexual health, and had gone to a lecture, but clearly hadn't learnt anything about sexually transmitted infections (STIs). He didn't know anything about the common antibiotics used, even though most of them are used in general medicine and surgery all the time. His body language was odd, seeming more interested in the floor than the patients. He didn't lean forward at interesting parts of the consultation, and he wasn't really listening – whenever he was invited to comment on what the patient had said he looked shocked and asked the patient to repeat.

He was basically just attending to get a tick in his logbook, and that is all that he got out of the session. It became easier, even for someone as passionate about teaching as the clinician involved, just to leave him sitting in the corner. A lengthy discussion after the clinic identified that he really didn't want to be a doctor.

Perhaps this seems like an extreme example; in actual fact it is relatively common for students not to engage in outpatient clinics.

If this student had read about two antibiotics and read just a couple of patient information leaflets before attending, then the student, the tutor and the patients would have had a much more productive and enjoyable experience. You will find plenty of other examples throughout the book, embedded in many of the submissions, but we have tried to cluster some here to highlight the point.

86. Why do some students get all the luck?

Some students get lots of teaching and always seem busy, whilst others don't. Some students tend to 'get noticed' (in a good way) whilst others seem invisible to the clinicians, or tend to get noticed in a less positive way.

Start a page in your notebook noting down the behaviours that the 'keener' students exhibit. Consider the wider aspects of their behaviour including body language, etc. Perhaps even interview them about their approach. You are likely to identify some simple strategies that would be easy to adopt.

Dason Evans, Doctor and Author

Taking it a step further

Think about expanding this task, to sample more widely and gain a consensus on what the most useful strategies are. Consider asking clinical teachers how they would describe a keen student compared with a less keen student. There are plenty of different approaches that you could use to sample more widely; you could even think of doing this as a medical education project.

87. Motivate your teachers

There are many simple things that you can do to demonstrate your keenness, as demonstrated by the submissions below.

If you are sitting around doing nothing on the ward, then grab a patient X-ray and stick it on a light box. Not only will this improve your knowledge of X-rays and how to interpret them but usually a doctor will stop and ask what you see, and you will then get a tutorial on the X-ray as well.

Donna Pilkington, Medical Student, UK

After a ward round the PRHOs do 'jobs', e.g. take blood, cannulate, arrange X-rays, etc. It is very worthwhile to shadow the PRHOs as they do these because they will (if you ask politely!) allow students to help carry out these procedures or at the very least explain how they are done. This is useful practice for procedural skills in the OSCE. You can also obtain feedback from the PRHOs and they can tell you what things you are doing right/wrong.

Sometimes after a ward round the whole team quickly seems to disappear somewhere leaving the students with nothing to do until lunch. The PRHOs usually go for a coffee break and students should ask them if they can join them. The PRHOs will be impressed by this as they will think that these students are keen and hence will be more willing to teach and explain things. It is also useful to shadow the PRHOs as much as possible because the students will be doing the same thing themselves soon.

Ravi Agarwal, Medical Student, UK

88. Preparing for surgery

I love surgery ... surgical patients are sometimes like candy and being allowed to scrub in during a surgery is one thing I love. There is the story of two of my colleagues being thrown out of surgery on their ears having not known anything about the patient and not knowing basic anatomy. Though unfortunate for them, we all learnt a valuable lesson. Clerk your patients before surgery — this is not as time-consuming as I once thought and takes 5 minutes to familiarise yourself with the appropriate anatomy. Once in surgery, you will shine in front of your consultant and you may even be taught on anatomy in its best form.

Laura Geddes, Medical Student, UK

Taking it a step further

How about compiling a common list of questions that surgeons ask in theatre (such as the anatomy of the anterior abdominal wall, and 'How do I know this is the ureter?', etc). You will find that many of the same things keep coming up time and time again.

Theme: finding other teachers

Background

This book has an emphasis on improving learning, and one way (but by no means the only way) of doing this is to widen the range of people who might teach you. Throughout the other sections of this book there are numerous submissions suggesting 'going elsewhere', which we draw together in this theme to highlight the huge variety that hospitals have to offer.

We have mentioned elsewhere (Task 92) that there is no guarantee that these other people will agree to teach you, but others have been successful. So, if you ask politely, what could be the worst that happens? It is worth knowing that some parts of the hospital rarely have students attached to them, and enthusiastic teachers in these locations yearn for a keen student to appear.

Remember, of course, that out of sight is out of mind. If you are attached to one team and you go off on a quiet day to join the ECG technicians (for example Task 43), then if your team know where you are, they will probably be impressed. If they do not know where you are, they will assume that you are skiving.

Requirements

All you need is a hospital, some 'cheek and charm' and a thick skin for the times that you get rejected. You will find some strategies for asking that work better than others – asking a radiologist to teach you anatomy may be less successful than asking him or her to talk you through the structures on a chest radiograph, for example.

Do not forget to ask permission from anyone who might be relevant, and, as always, ensure that the patients are able to give you fully informed consent.

Phlebotomy department tasks

Submissions include going to the phlebotomy department and asking to take blood and shadowing the phlebotomists on the wards (Task 44).

Radiology department tasks

Various submissions highlighting the role of the radiology department in teaching anatomy, in getting to 'know about' some of the procedures that they perform, data interpretation, and even in providing opportunities for practising practical procedures like cannulation (Tasks 70, 73, 83 and 85).

MAU and A&E tasks

Both the medical assessment unit (MAU), or acute admitting ward, and the accident and emergency department (A&E) will usually provide plenty of opportunities for practical procedures, history taking, physical examination (Task 46).

Anaesthetists' tasks

Anaesthetists have quite varied jobs, involving anaesthetising patients, looking after intensive therapy units (ITUs), perioperative care and a wide range of other things. They are generally relaxed people, keen to teach, who rarely have students. They know a lot of head and neck anatomy, a huge amount of physiology, and rely on a strong understanding of basic pharmacology and pharmacodynamics to enable them to anaesthetise patients safely. They therefore make a fantastic resource! (Tasks 45 and 46).

Many hospitals will have a dedicated pain team, who usually have a role in advising on the management of patients in pain, and also specifically teaching about pain management – important for all doctors (Task 63).

Other ward and other ward-round tasks

There is usually nothing to stop you from looking further afield from the ward to which you are attached; just make sure that your team know where you are, that you explain your presence to the nurses and doctors in the new location, and that you are not stepping on other students' toes. Examples include the cardiology ward for patients with murmurs, the elderly care or rehabilitation wards for patients with neurological signs, and going to other wards simply to motivate yourself, or in search of clinicians with an excellent reputation for teaching

Outpatient clinic tasks

Outpatient departments provide a wide variety of specialty and generalist clinics. What better way to practise examination of patients with hernia, for example, than in a dedicated hernia clinic? Along a similar line, don't forget day-case surgery lists.

Other professional tasks

Interprofessional education is discussed in Section 6, and runs through many different submissions in this book. Examples include the thrombolysis nurse, ward pharmacist, other specialist nurses, ECG technicians and phlebotomists.

Section 9
EFFECTIVENESS AND EFFICIENCY

Be sure you put your feet in the right place, then stand firm.

Abraham Lincoln

Introduction

If you are reading this book from start to finish, you will have realised by now that most of the sections (and indeed many of the themes) overlap – similar to a rather complex Venn diagram. This is particularly true of this section: building your effectiveness and efficiency is one of the key themes of this book.

Making learning fun (and indeed making work fun) is crucially important. Think for a second of a topic that you were motivated to learn – how easy it was to remember everything – and contrast this with a topic for which you didn't feel motivated. You will have had friends who were motivated in your least favourite topic – the difference is in the motivation, not the topic. Intrinsic motivation and interest are the key to learning. The concept of positive spirals is interesting, and one that you will see implicitly throughout this book; this concept states that you can deliberately influence your own motivation. Imagine, for example, that you find liver disease a frustrating and dull topic. You have never got to grips with it, there just seems too much to learn and you find yourself staring at the pages. There are a number of actions that you can take:

1. Break it down into small steps

2. Arrange to attend the viral hepatitis clinic

3. Pencil in a few hours to learn about hepatitis B, and particularly the national guidelines and what the various blood test results mean.

During the clinic you should find an opportunity to ask questions and get the most out of the clinicians. The respect that you get as a student who seems interested will be great for your motivation and will encourage you to learn more (and the clinicians will be keen to teach you more too!). That night you will look up more about hepatitis B and we guarantee that it will have become much easier to remember. Motivated students get more from teaching and we hope that this section demonstrates how you can actively manage your motivation, and as a result find learning easier and gain more from teaching.

101 Things to Do with Spare Moments on the Ward, First Edition. Dason E Evans, Nakul Gamanlal Patel.
© 2012 Dason E Evans and Nakul Gamanlal Patel. Published 2012 by Blackwell Publishing Ltd.

This section includes submissions and ideas about how to manage your own motivation and it includes some of the more amusing submissions to hopefully put a smile on your face on those days when things seem a little grim. We have also included some thoughts on planning for your career, including research and audits. The first 2 years as a doctor will involve undertaking a large amount of administration and we have included some top tips at the end of this section to help you think now about learning those organisational skills while still a medical student.

Theme: knowing your own motivation

As we discussed in the introduction, knowing what motivates you and actively managing it is a key to learning. This is not as easy as it may seem, because different medical students are motivated by different aspects of their role. For some it is about caring for others, for others it is a diagnostic challenge, and others like to feel useful and part of a team. Some are motivated by seeing that they are learning, others by seeing that they are doing. Do you know what motivates you?

89. Doing things that motivate you

At times when there is nothing to do in the ward I'm allocated to, I try to go to another ward that has patients in an area of medicine of my own interest (neurology for me) and ask staff for interesting patients with interesting histories or signs to expand upon my learning opportunities.

Ali Al-Iami, Medical Student, UK

90. Feeding patients

Go along during meal times and ask the nurses if there are any patients who require help with feeding. Whether it is actively feeding the patient or just sitting with them to give them company and encouragement, it's a great feeling to be actually doing something worthwhile, and you'll probably get the patient's story too.

Laura Cohen, Medical Student, UK

Authors' note: helping patients feed can be an advanced nursing skill, in terms of both helping patients avoid aspiration and, just as importantly, helping patients to maintain dignity despite their dependence. If you are uncertain, or if the patient has significant dysphagia, ask the nurses or physiotherapists for advice.

91. What have I done today?

Okay so you're bored on the wards and, more than this, feeling useless. A simple method of rectifying this; make a mental list of all the useful things that you have done today and who has benefitted. Think about patients (e.g. taking the time to check on a patient's wellbeing — making them feel cared for), think about your firm (e.g. took blood for your house officer — allowing them to get on with something more pressing), think about the whole medical team (e.g. talking to the stoma nurse about a patient who is having difficulties emptying a bag — alerting him/her to a patient's need) and think about what you have learned (e.g. that spare moment you spent reading Kumar and Clark about xeroderma pigmentosum because your consultant mentioned it).

Soon enough you realise that you have achieved a lot today — and even that the small tasks make a difference to a patient or colleague and certainly your own learning. Furthermore, if you have a gap in the list (e.g. you have done nothing for your firm today, or you have not checked up on that patient you clerked) then you have just found something to do!

So there you have it — a useful confidence-boosting exercise!

Saleem Farooqui, Medical Student, UK

While on ward rounds and if nobody is talking to you and you feel like a spare wheel, take the time to help your F1/F2. Learn how to take notes and ask them if they wouldn't mind if you helped write them, or take over the use of the computer. Getting patient's blood results and X-rays could be your thing to do while the team are discussing the patient. This will save time during the ward round and you can try to interpret the results before showing the rest of the team to see what they come up with. If you therefore have a question on what you're looking at, you can ask them while they are looking at it.

This was definitely a skill that I learnt late on during my clinical year. I found I learnt more, I felt useful on ward rounds and that I was part of the team.

Kayur Patel, Medical Student, UK

92. Managing demotivating influences

As much as it is important to know what motivates you, it is also important to know what demotivates you.

We select a professor, mentor, instructor... and one of us mimics that person exactly.

Then we choose the case which the doctor would discuss with us the following day in the round... The student who plays the doctor guesses almost all the questions the doctor would ask... and the flaws he is going to pick for us and even the bitter criticism we are going to receive from him during the round. It was a great fun when most of our predictions come true and helped us absorb any bitter words; it even brought us to laughter... those are days we will never forget.

It is the 'GUESS GAME'.

Professor Omayma Aly, Doctor, Egypt

This exercise not only provides armour against the verbal onslaught of some of your less constructive tutors, but it also has additional benefits. It may give you some insights as to what is behind the 'bitter criticisms' – usually it is a misguided attempt to encourage you to learn; they really believe that intimidation is a good teaching tool! This will be particularly useful for some of the more timid medical students.

Taking it a step further

Role play being the most arrogant clinician whom you have come across – make sure that you are with friends and will not be observed. Pay particular attention to your body language: shoulders, arms, angle of head on the body; ask your colleagues for feedback. You will notice something strange happening – that you begin to feel more confident. Use this exercise to reflect on how you might appear more confident (without becoming the most arrogant clinician that you have ever met!).

Theme: fun and flippant suggestions

There have been numerous flippant submissions for the book, and we have included some of the very best here. We felt it important to include these 'fun' suggestions within a book on learning to represent an even work–life balance. If you don't agree, just look at what these well-known individuals have to say on it:

Almost all creativity involves purposeful play.

Abraham Maslow

Fun is at the core of the way I like to do business and it has been the key to everything I've done from the outset. More than any other element, fun is the secret of Virgin's success.

Richard Branson

He who does not get fun and enjoyment out of every day … needs to reorganize his life.

George Matthew Adams

We suspect that those who have suggested fun and flippant 'things' to do are more aware of their own energy levels, and have made suggestions that are likely to boost enthusiasm by either re-enacting them or simply a quiet read and a chuckle at a low moment.

We have mentioned professional boundaries before, and 'having a laugh' while remaining professional can be a particular challenge. It is worth remembering that doctors are human and are allowed to have fun. We have included suggestions that we think are appropriately professional, although some of them might come close to the boundary. Perhaps when you read through this section, you could spare a moment to think about whether each suggestion would be appropriate for you, or for a colleague, and what might make it more appropriate and what might make it unacceptable.

93. Get some exercise

Kids (and me) get bored easily. Having just finished a paeds firm, I discovered the best way to bond with children is to endanger their lives and push them at speed around the ward on desk chairs.

The parents love it, it's good exercise and it made my consultant smile (which is rare).

The louder they scream, the more fun they are having.

Andrew Pelham, Medical Student, UK

This is more of a light-hearted and, well, immature time filler. I myself am a first year medical student but by having a parent in the medical profession I have heard about this 'sport'. Not sure if it's widely done, so thought I'd mention it anyway.

The setting I heard about it in was a quiet A&E department during the middle of the night. The specific layout of the ward had a workstation in the centre that led to circular shape ward. It would work just as well in a straight ward I'm sure.

Basically it's the 'sport' of wheelchair racing. I would imagine you could play it two ways. Either singly, and racing other staff, or, if the wheelchair was hard to move by yourself, having a partner to push you.

Race around or down the ward and the first to finish wins. With a ward with lots of staff and time on their hands I presume a little tournament could be drawn up! (In some cases I'd imagine patients might like to play!)

Andrew Smith, Medical Student, UK

Both of these suggestions might make the health and safety officers nervous; Andrew Pelham's inclusion of the parents and consultant demonstrates his awareness of these issues.

Dance round a drip stand.

Ruth Bird, Medical Student, UK

94. Food glorious food

Find the doctors' mess for free toast. Toast is a food group in itself and sustains life very well.

Ruth Bird, Medical Student, UK

Feel a bit faint because you neglected to eat breakfast because the shop was shut because you had to leave so early to be in so there was no milk for cereal? So neatly sneak away from the ward round then on the stairs on the way to the canteen have a sit down to regain yourself and be accosted by some resus man who insists on wheeling you to A&E for extensive tests. Result: you eat a sandwich and are fine. Not exactly the art of modern medicine but it passes the time.

Anonymous Medical Student, UK

Taking it a step further

In every hospital there is a 'safe haven' ward – one where the junior doctors can go when life is getting too much, a ward where the nurses will spot a forlorn looking doctor, whisk them into a chair, perhaps answer their bleep for them for 5 minutes and maybe even crack open the secret drawer that contains expensive biscuits and really decent coffee. When covering these wards, junior doctors will 'find' themselves popping in to check that all is ok, and just perhaps stop for a slice of toast. After a brief 5-minute break, of course, they become far more productive.

Aim to locate one or two of these oases in every hospital to which you are attached. With practice you will find them easier to spot, a skill that you will really appreciate later on in your career.

---

95. Books and the arts

Read House of God so as to become more aware just what your chosen career entails.

Ruth Bird, Medical Student, UK

You will find plenty of books to read that will change your perspective on medicine. *House of God*, by Samuel Shem, gives a harsh and cynical look at the practice of medicine in the USA. If you read this book, consider how it has changed the way that you view medicine and patients – some doctors seem to become a little less humane after reading it.

Other titles that might have a more positive impact on your thoughts about medicine and about patients include:

- *The Diving-Bell and the Butterfly* by Jean-Dominique Bauby
- *The Spirit Catches You and You Fall Down: A Hmong child, her American doctors and the collision of two cultures* by Anne Fadiman
- *To The Wedding* by John Berger
- *Illness as Metaphor* and *AIDS and Its Metaphors* by Susan Sontag
- *The Story of San Michele* by Axel Munthe

Several of the journals and many websites have produced lists of recommended 'non-medical' books for medical students, and there have been research papers on the value of reading such texts, e.g. Hampshire and Avery (2001). There are also lists of films relevant to medicine.

Why not interview your peers and your tutors about relevant books from the classics?

Theme: never too early to think about your future

In those spare moments, there are plenty of opportunities to think about your future career, plan ways of enhancing your CV and, more importantly, enhancing your experience and understanding of the different specialties (we consider general practice to be one of the medical specialties). This theme includes suggestions about looking forward and preparing for the future.

96. Never too early to think about your future

Read some old elective reports. These are usually kept in your medical school library. This will give you some ideas on how to go about arranging your elective early and also help to focus you on what you want to achieve from your elective experience. Believe me, this will reduce stress later on in the year.

Alison Bradley, Medical Student, UK

For those of you who are keen to do some extra work, make enquiries within departments as to whether any of the consultants have any ideas for audits they would like carried out. This will fill up all those half-hour- and odd hour-long brakes you might find you have during the day. It also looks good on a CV and will get you known as a keen student within the department.

Alison Bradley, Medical Student, UK

Theme: organisation and efficiency

Background

I'm a great believer in luck, and I find the harder I work the more I have of it.
Thomas Jefferson

This section aims to demonstrate a very basic relationship that you may find useful for developing effectiveness and efficiency in your working life.

Organised → Familiarity → Efficiency → Success

To explain this flowchart with an example, when learning to take bloods, the best way to begin is to **organise** your equipment, i.e. tourniquet, cannulas, blood bottles, antiseptic wipe, sharps bin, vacutainer. This will prevent you from having to stop and look for things during the procedure, which can make you come across as a novice.

Repetition of the procedure will allow you to develop **familiarity**. This in turn will make you more **efficient** at the task in hand, which will lead you to become more **successful** at your work.

Requirements

It is solely up to you to be organised and efficient. You need to go to the ward each day with an open mind and open eyes! Go with a positive attitude and intention of coming away having learnt at least one thing. This way you will see and seize any opportunities present, grabbing them eagerly with both hands.

In summary, the requirements for this section are the heart of the entire book. You need to have a **willingness** to learn the very basics. Be **proactive**; if you are bored and have nothing to do, find a nurse to shadow, asking questions, look through a patient's record and understand the drugs that the patient is on and why, and maybe consider any interactions/contraindications. These are just a few examples of time well spent.

Slowly, all the practical knowledge that you gain will be invaluable. You will tend to remember this more profoundly than reading a textbook, because you will relate a real-life patient to a problem or drug!

As the saying goes, 'drop by drop, the ocean is formed'; similarly you will find that continually being organised, grabbing opportunities and being efficient with any free time on the ward will result in a quick escalation of your knowledge base. This in turn will make you more efficient, resulting in a less stressful and easier life. Above all it will boost your confidence very quickly!

97. Signing up for sessions

If you are organised half the battle is won.

In Homerton, students are able to sign up to phlebotomy sessions with phlebotomy staff, where they are given a chance to practise on a dummy arm, and then on patients the staff would deem to be easier to take blood from. This gives students a chance to become confident in taking blood from real people. It is very useful, and sessions only last an hour. It is something useful to do when you are bored!

Debi Dasgupta, Medical Student, UK

So, if you were organised, you would have signed up for these phlebotomy sessions with the phlebotomy staff immediately; this would mean you were ahead of your peers. You would have attended these sessions and practised on dummy arms, going on to patients. By practising more and more you will have become efficient at carrying out this core skill. Consequently, when at last you qualify and are a junior doctor, and you are instructed to carry out this procedure on x number of patients, you would already feel familiar and confident to do so very efficiently. This would result in a successful task completed.

Taking it a step further

If we were to take the above task one step further, why not be the leader/organiser and take this idea forward:

Set up a 'sign-up phlebotomy session' at your hospital in conjunction with the phlebotomy service.

Meera Patel, Dentist and Author, UK

98. Ready to learn the basics

To know whether the bed is ready for the next patient, you need to know the hospital protocol and cross-infection procedures. You should never feel too small to help clean up and decontaminate empty beds; in fact by doing so, not only will you win nurses in your favour but at the same time you will solidify the fundamental principles in cross-infection control. Go with an open mind and ready to learn the basic procedures, and work yourself up. This core knowledge will help you become wiser, organised and efficient. This also links back to the other themes in this section and Section 6 – 'being curious' applies far more widely than just to cleaning beds.

Clean up and decontaminate empty patient beds.

Indrajith Kowarthanan, Medical Student, UK

Feeling in the way?

Do you sometimes feel like you are getting in the way? You are not the only one to have experienced this. Instead of tottering about on the ward, be efficient with your time.

Get the PRHO to bleep the diabetes nurse and see if she is free. If she is busy ask if you can shadow her and learn about diabetes management. Alternatively, if she is free she can spend time teaching about it!

This is useful when the team are busy and you feel 'in the way'. Especially because you learn about conservative control, all the types of insulins, sliding scales in hospitals, etc. A good morning well spent!

Nabila Salahuddin, Medical Student, UK

Using this sort of opportunity and showing that you are forthcoming and keen can generate positive energy. The nurses feel a boost of confidence and this will result in a great teaching opportunity – a win–win situation for all!

Observational learning

Observational learning is an invaluable tool for avoiding mistakes made by others, alongside learning successful skills that others have learnt through years of practical experience. Put yourselves in their shoes and think about how you would have dealt with the same situation/problem.

As we have already considered observing your seniors interacting with nursing staff, why not take it further by observing the bigger picture.

When there is 'nothing to do' on the ward, students could observe how other people work and how they are organised.

Students could try to think how would they do the tasks that they are observing and if there is better way of doing them (including communication, organisational, time management, clinical or any other skills) and if there is any way they would be able to improve the observed skill/action when they find themselves in similar situation(s).

Natasa Perovic, CELT, UK

99. Clues to spot learning

Whenever you are around a patient, be a detective and investigate for signs to uncover what condition(s) the patient has. This could be done using a multitude of clues such as bedside items, equipment around the patient, and the drug chart. There are a lot of cues that can help you formulate a diagnosis; the more experience you gain the better you will become.

This is yet another technique that will allow you to make efficient use of your time.

When examining the patient we see a lot of tubing, different types of Venflons and other related material. Most of the time we question why they choose that colour of Venflon and not another, why they are using that type of infusion or why some patients have an oddly yellow-coloured IV infusion bag. Most of these things can be clearly learnt by spending just about 30 minutes in the ward equipment room. Here one can check out the different Venflon sizes and the different stuff one finds next to a patient. Also the different types of infusions present.

This exercise only takes a few minutes, yet it saves a lot of questioning time during ward rounds or helps a lot during the practical exam since it might indicate certain unique features. If a patient has a yellow IV infusion bag attached to his Venflon, it might well be that he has vitamin supplements and thus can help in certain pathological identification. Also by knowing the Venflon colour one can see if it is a normal Venflon or one to attach infusions to, or one inserted in an artery for quick ABGs. Also, different types of vacuum bottles, why they have that distinct rim colour and their use.

Possibly, one can ask a nurse to help out to identify the use of an object or to show how the unit works such as heparin continuous infusion pumps.

Karl Cutajar, Medical Student, Malta

Taking it a step further

There will be many occasions where you feel as though you have nothing to do and yet you are not allowed to leave the ward. Well what a fantastic chance to analyse existing patients' records and data. You can ask numerous questions relating to every aspect of the history taken, investigations carried out, provisional diagnoses given, treatment carried out and prognosis – interesting, right?

The student could have a look at the existing data (all kind of documents, lab results, X-rays, etc.) about a patient (he/she knows or not) and try to reflect on the following questions:

- Do I understand all medical terms?
  If not, look them up
- Do I understand why the doctor came up with the actual diagnosis?
  If yes, list all the arguments you know which speak for
  If no, write down your doubts and where you lost the track (discuss it, if possible, with a peer student or your supervisor at the wards)
- Would I add something else? (Other tests, etc?)
  If yes, list them and why you think they might be useful
- Which is the structure of a clear report?
  List the titles of the structure (e.g. present problem [symptoms, signs], history, test done, etc.)

Martina Michels, Physiotherapist, UK

Work with your friends and look at each patient from afar. Then, guess what conditions they may suffer with, justifying this with evidence from peripheral paraphernalia around the bed or visual physical signs. The loser buys lunch.

Gaman Patel, Businessman, UK

Preparing for the future

If there are any basic clinical procedures that you feel incompetent doing, enquire about opportunities available to allow for you to go in, learn and practise under supervision.

Join the cannulation or phlebotomy team on their rounds. Phlebs tend to do early morning; the cannulation team — at my hospital at least — hold bleeps and are on call 8–8pm. You can stay with them to do just one cannula/bloods or spend up to a whole day depending on how much time you have free/your level of confidence doing it. It is a great idea to really boost your confidence and will make your first few weeks at work so much easier and less stressful if you are quick and efficient and not daunted by blood taking/cannulation when on call for the wards. Plus your team will love you!

Catherine Culley, Doctor, UK

Taking it a step further

If you are unclear or not confident about carrying out a 12-lead ECG find a suitable trained nurse to teach you and then let you do it. Similarly, if you feel incompetent about placing chest drains, why not find a doctor who is willing to teach you and then let you place them under supervision until you feel competent. This can be practised with all procedures.

See also

Sections 4 and 6.

---

100. GP receptionist

It is important for you to realise that you can take your organisational and time management skills and apply them to any situation, e.g. you can apply them to your general practice placements as shown in the example below.

Students have time between seeing patients in general practice. Instead of waiting for the next patient to arrive they could go and see if a receptionist is free to talk. The theme could be varied like how does the receptionist decide how urgent an appointment is? What is the receptionist's view on who deserves an appointment? The receptionist's view on how to match patients to doctors (in a multi-doctor practice).

As a next step the student might try to man the appointment telephone line for an hour.

The theme could be changed to repeat prescriptions, nurse appointments — an endless number of topics.

Martin Mueller, Doctor, UK

Sit down with the receptionist and observe all the work he or she is carrying out.

Asil Tahir, Medical Student, UK

Reference

Hampshire AJ, Avery AJ (2001). What can students learn from studying medicine in literature? *Med Educ* **35**:687–90.

Section 10
OVER TO YOU

Task 101

Some readers will have noticed that this book is called '101 things ...' and yet there are only 100 core, highlighted, numbered suggestions (or tasks). This is deliberate. The 101st suggestion/task is blank. This book has two aims. The first is simple – to share some ideas on how to make better use of the clinical environment as a learning environment. The second is to try to help you to spot other ideas for yourself, try them out, see which ones work, which don't, and to share this with other people; you will have noticed this as a thread running throughout the whole of the book.

> Choose your five best original ideas for 'things to do' in spare moments by trying them out with peers and colleagues – then submit them to share with others at **www.101things.org**.

101 Things to Do with Spare Moments on the Ward, First Edition. Dason E Evans, Nakul Gamanlal Patel.
© 2012 Dason E Evans and Nakul Gamanlal Patel. Published 2012 by Blackwell Publishing Ltd.

Index

101 Things to Do with Spare Moments on the Ward, First Edition. Dason E Evans, Nakul Gamanlal Patel.
© 2012 Dason E Evans and Nakul Gamanlal Patel. Published 2012 by Blackwell Publishing Ltd.

Keep up with critical fields

Would you like to receive up-to-date information on our books, journals and databases in the areas that interest you, direct to your mailbox?

Join the **Wiley e-mail service** - a convenient way to receive updates and exclusive discount offers on products from us.

Simply visit **www.wiley.com/email** and register online

We won't bombard you with emails and we'll only email you with information that's relevant to you. We will ALWAYS respect your e-mail privacy and NEVER sell, rent, or exchange your e-mail address to any outside company. Full details on our privacy policy can be found online.

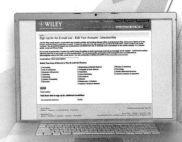

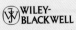